R U N A W A Y
E A T I N G

RUNAWAY EATING

The 8-Point Plan to Conquer
Adult Food and Weight Obsessions

CYNTHIA M. BULIK, Ph.D.,
AND NADINE TAYLOR, M.S., R.D.

RODALE

© 2005 by Cynthia M. Bulik, Ph.D., and Nadine Taylor, M.S., R.D.

Printed in the United States of America
Rodale Inc. makes every effort to use acid-free ⊗, recycled paper ♻.

Book design by UGD/DesignWorks

Illustrations by Karen Kuchar

Library of Congress Cataloging-in-Publication Data

Bulik, Cynthia M.
    Runaway eating : the 8-point plan to conquer adult food and weight obsessions / Cynthia M. Bulik and Nadine Taylor.
       p.   cm.
    Includes bibliographical references and index.
    ISBN-13 978–1–59486–038–6 paperback
    ISBN-10 1–59486–038–6 paperback
    1. Eating disorders in women—Treatment. 2. Eating disorders in women—Psychological aspects. 3. Middle-aged women—Health and hygiene. I. Taylor, Nadine. II. Title.
RC552.E18B84 2005
616.85'26—dc22   2004022477

Distributed to the trade by Holtzbrinck Publishers

2 4 6 8 10 9 7 5 3   paperback

For Pat, Brendan, Emily, and Natalie, around whom my world revolves.

—C. B.

For my parents, Jay and Nina Taylor, who would have been proud.

—N. T.

Contents

An Epidemic of Food Misuse

"It seems like my whole life revolves around serving the needs of others—my kids, my boss, my husband, you name it! Everyone wants a piece of me, and lately I've been waking up in a panic in the middle of the night wondering how I'm going to get it all done. My life is out of control and, unfortunately, so is my eating. When I finally get a few moments alone, I like to close the blinds and bury myself in a half gallon of ice cream. Only then can I feel the anxiety melt away."

—Dawnette, age 37

Have you ever eaten half a chocolate cake, then felt terrible about yourself? Do you feel that your eating habits are out of control? Have you been on some form of a diet for as long as you can remember? Do you hate your weight, your shape, or your body in general to the point where you cringe whenever you look in a mirror, try on clothes, or see pictures of yourself? Is having a body that's slim, trim, and sexy still incredibly important to you, even though you're no longer in your twenties? Do you run away from your problems by indulging in your favorite comfort foods? If you answered yes to any of these questions, then this book is for you.

We women are caught in the throes of a love/hate relationship with food. Currently, 62 percent of American women are overweight or obese (about two-thirds of us!), up from 42 percent in 1976. Even more frightening is the fact that almost half of today's overweight women fall into the obese category. Since 1976, overweight among women has increased by 50 percent, while the rate of obesity has actually doubled. (And men aren't doing much better.)

These statistics are certainly indications of an epidemic of food misuse going on right under our noses. But even as we yield to the siren call of food, we find ourselves furious for doing so. We loathe every extra pound of fat and beat ourselves up about it, get depressed, or work like crazy to get rid of it. Yet no matter what we do to make ourselves feel better about our bodies, we're rarely happy with the results. According to the National Eating Disorders Association, 80 percent of American women are dissatisfied with their bodies. That means that only one woman in five actually thinks her body is okay. Not surprisingly, this dissatisfaction translates into a huge market for diets, with some $40 billion spent in the United States every year on dieting and diet-related products.

Unfortunately, in spite of all the time, effort, and money invested in these diets, the failure rate is nothing short of spectacular. A full 90 to 95 percent of dieters end up regaining the weight they lost (and often more) within 5 years. This isn't surprising, because diets tend to slow down the body's metabolism, making it much easier to pile on pounds. And muscle tissue that was lost while dieting tends to be replaced with fat, resulting in a higher percentage of body fat than ever before. Further, despite our good intentions, we may be damaging our health as a result of all this dieting. Many of the popular fad diets are nutritionally unbalanced, increasing the risk for vitamin and mineral deficiencies and possibly the risk for heart attack and stroke. So we who are unhappy with our bodies find ourselves caught in a dilemma: We can bounce from stuffing to starving and back again, sacrificing our physical and mental health in pursuit of an "acceptable" body. Or we can simply give up and try to live with our overweight, believing that we really can't do much about it. Of course, neither one is a satisfactory solution.

Even worse, the underlying problem—that the vast majority of us, whether thin or fat, dieting or not, have major issues with food—remains completely ignored. We use food to fight boredom, depression, anxiety, and anger; to ease stress; to reward ourselves; and to mask emotional emptiness—all of which have nothing to do with nourishing the body.

Most of us don't have the symptoms of a clinically defined eating disorder, such as anorexia nervosa or bulimia nervosa, but we'd be hard-pressed to deny that our relationships with food and our own bodies are often unhealthy. In fact, a tremendous number of us have out-of-control, "runaway" eating behaviors. And often, these behaviors are the result of our using food to run away from our problems. We've dubbed this double "runaway" problem *Runaway Eating*. You can think of it as a kind of pre–eating disorder. Although the driving forces behind both Runaway Eating and clinically defined eating disorders are basically the same, the symptoms aren't as severe or frequent for a Runaway Eater. But no matter how mild the symptoms might be, the defining features of Runaway Eating are the *consistent use of food or food-related behaviors (such as purging or exercising excessively) to deal with unpleasant feelings* and *feeling that these behaviors are out of control.* Left untreated, Runaway Eating can damage your health, happiness, self-esteem, and relationships, and the quality of your life.

Until now, the large and growing population of Runaway

Eaters has been unidentified and untreated, because most of us don't fit any standard diagnostic criteria. Or we may feel too embarrassed to ask for help, because we believe that these are problems we should be able to control. We may even dismiss the severity of our problems, believing that out-of-control eating or fasting is the domain of teenagers, not grown women. Whatever the reason, Runaway Eating runs rampant throughout our society, particularly during the super-stressful midlife years when hormone fluctuations, family responsibilities, financial pressures, and other troubles typically reach a peak. Eating and eating-related behaviors offer a tempting escape, whether the escape takes the form of restrictive dieting, bingeing, excessive exercise, bingeing and purging, or just stuffing down unwanted emotions with chocolate cream pie. But this "solution" is no solution.

HOPE AND HELP FOR RUNAWAY EATERS

The good news is that you can get a handle on Runaway Eating and banish it from your life forever. In this book, we explain the three forms of Runaway Eating and lay out a comprehensive self-treatment program to help you identify and solve the problems behind your unhealthy relationship with food. You'll discover how and why your Runaway Eating evolved, and learn how these behaviors serve a specific nonfood function in your life. In addition, you'll find out how to:

- Identify the situations that set off your Runaway Eating cycle
- Avoid these triggers, nip them in the bud, or handle them in a more positive way

- Think about food and weight in completely new, healthy ways
- Eat regularly, without letting your emotions determine when, how, or what you eat
- Uncover the connection between your eating habits and your thoughts, feelings, and behaviors
- Challenge your Thought Myths and replace them with healthier alternatives
- Balance bad moods without the use of food
- Release and reduce stress, and manage anxiety
- Ease the depression that can drive Runaway Eating
- Effectively manage menopausal and perimenopausal symptoms
- Conquer perfectionism
- Avoid relapse

As a clinical psychologist with more than 20 years' experience in treating patients with eating disorders, and a registered dietitian who has worked with people who have eating disorders, we have combined our knowledge and experience to bring you the latest information on problematic eating from both the psychological and nutritional perspectives. The case histories and personal experiences you will read in this book are taken from our lectures, workshops, and discussions with patients and families. (In addition, Nadine has had personal experience with a mild form of an eating disorder, as detailed in "My Story" on page xiv.) Using these examples and writing in simple, clear, nontechnical language, we'll explain the real reasons that so many midlife women suffer from out-of-control eating and what to do about it. We offer millions of Runaway Eaters a safe and sane approach to overcoming

MY STORY

In my mid- to late twenties, during the late 1970s era of "You can never be too thin or too rich," I became a Runaway Eater. Single, about 20 pounds overweight, somewhat depressed, and convinced that my ticket to happiness lay in looking as good as possible, I tried diet after diet. But the diets just made me want to eat. They also made me nervous, down on myself, and obsessed with my weight—I actually had a sign pasted above my desk that read, "All beautiful women are thin." But no matter how determined I was, I could never stay on a diet for more than a couple of days. And every so often, I'd start eating like crazy, unable to stop myself.

My Runaway Eating episodes occurred about every 3 months over a couple of years, not enough to qualify as bona fide bulimia. But the cause and effect was much the same. Standing in front of my refrigerator, feeling nervous, lonely, or just plain tired of holding myself in, I'd allow myself to eat a little bit of something that was off my diet, like an extra carton of yogurt or a big spoonful of peanut butter. Of course, that was never satisfying enough, so I'd progress to a little squiggle of cake, which then became a bigger piece, which eventually became half the cake.

At some point, I'd realize that I had gone too far and the only "solution" was to throw up and rid myself of all those calories. And if I was going to throw it all up anyway, why not just completely let go and eat whatever I wanted?

problem eating, avoiding pathological dieting, eating healthfully, and avoiding relapse.

This book is for the millions of people who suffer from out-of-control eating behaviors ranging from mild to severe, whether only occasionally or every day of their lives. Runaway Eaters are people who otherwise appear to be normal and in control of their lives, yet who have unhealthy relationships with food or their

Then came the food free-for-all—I'd stuff down anything I could find that was sweet or starchy, until my stomach couldn't hold another bite. Although I still didn't feel satisfied, it was such a relief to stop restricting! Of course, getting rid of it was a chore—and quite a disgusting one—but sometimes afterward, I'd go right back to eating again and repeat the process. It was years before I realized that I was eating for reasons that had nothing to do with food.

My Runaway Eating ended when I finally decided to stop dieting and being a slave to my weight and my looks. I resolved to try to eat healthful foods and nourish my body, but if I really wanted a hot fudge sundae or some other treat, I'd have it without feeling guilty. I also had a few other rules: I never skipped a meal, I always ate something whenever I felt hungry, and I tried to stop eating the instant I felt full. To my great surprise, within 6 months my weight had stabilized at 8 pounds lower than it had been in years, and I completely lost the urge to binge.

Since that time (it's been more than 20 years), I have actually liked my body and the way it looks. (My weight fluctuates by plus or minus 5 pounds, but I never worry about it.) You couldn't get me near a diet, and I would never make myself throw up again, under any circumstances. Although Runaway Eating ruled my life for a while, I conquered it—and you can, too.

—Nadine Taylor

bodies that can interfere with personal relationships, threaten their quality of life, and set them up for future health problems. This book is for you, me, and the woman down the street—it's for everybody who wonders why she can't seem to get a handle on her eating problems and has decided to do something about it.

At last, Runaway Eaters can discover the tools they need to regain control of their eating, their bodies, and their lives.

Part One

UNDERSTANDING RUNAWAY EATING

CHAPTER 1

Not for Teenagers Only:
The Rise of Midlife Eating Problems

"Among the recent pressures on women, perhaps
none is more severe than linking femininity with
slimness and fitness. . . . Slim, trim, bright, beautiful,
and driven are now the standards set for the modern
middle-class woman . . ."

—James M. Mannon, *Measuring Up: The Performance
Ethic in American Culture*

Liz, a 45-year-old interior designer and mother of two young
children, began to use food to run away from the stresses in
her life just after her marriage fell apart. Within a period of about
6 months, her life turned upside down. Besides having to adjust
to being single again, Liz saw her workload double as she went
from a part-time to a full-time schedule, requiring her to hire a
live-in nanny. She found herself in the throes of a nasty custody
battle, her finances were in disarray, and both children began to
do poorly in school. Going from bad to worse, Liz's mother died,
and Liz herself began going through early menopause. Some days
she felt as if she was on an emotional roller coaster.

"Sometimes the only thing that can make me feel better is eating an entire box of chocolate-covered caramels," Liz admitted. But her Runaway Eating didn't stop there. When she felt particularly anxious or sad, she could eat 2 quarts of ice cream in one sitting, a dozen doughnuts on her way to work, or an entire jar of peanut butter by the spoonful. Her weight soared and she felt bloated and awful, but that didn't keep her from bingeing the next time.

"After I go on one of my eating jags, I'm always disgusted with myself, and I end up feeling even worse (make that a lot worse) than when I started," Liz sighed. "But still, I just can't seem to stop. . . ." In the course of trying to find comfort, distraction, solace, and satisfaction through food—in short, using food to run away from her problems—Liz found that her eating habits had run away with *her*.

Problematic eating has long been considered the almost exclusive territory of troubled teenage girls and young women. We've all read about Karen Carpenter's self-induced starvation and Princess Diana's bingeing and purging. We've heard dramatic stories about the high-achieving teenage girl who starves herself down to 60 pounds, the stressed-out college student who binges and purges 10 times a day, and the driven gymnast who works out 8 hours a day, then goes home and does a 90-minute high-speed session on her stationary bike. You might think, as Liz once did, that these destructive, dangerous behaviors are just kid stuff and that once you've safely passed through your twenties, you're immune from such traps.

Yet an invisible class of problem eaters has been quietly growing in recent years: women in their thirties, forties, fifties, and beyond. In the past 5 years, psychologists nationwide have noticed a startling rise in the number of midlife women seeking treatment for eating problems. In March 2003, the *New York Times* reported that the number of over-40 patients at the Remuda Ranch in Arizona, the nation's second-largest eating disorder treatment center, had more than doubled since 1997. A similar increase was seen at the Cornell Eating Disorders Program in White Plains, New York— with twice as many midlife women motivated to get help than there were 5 years earlier. Part of the increase may be due to the growing availability of such programs and a decrease in the shame associated with reaching out for help. But beyond that, more and more women are realizing that problematic eating is ruining their lives. Hard statistics reflecting the scope of midlife eating problems are difficult to come by, partly because most women don't seek help until their troubles become unbearable. We do know that of the 8 million Americans with bona fide eating disorders, a full 14 percent (more than 1 million people) are not teenagers. And surely this is only the tip of the iceberg. Full-blown eating disorders don't just suddenly appear out of nowhere; they develop gradually over a period of years or even decades. They also exist in degrees, ranging from very mild to very severe. Undoubtedly, millions of women suffer from the milder forms of disordered eating that can show up as occasional bouts of out-of-control eating, weight preoccupation, pathological dieting, bingeing, occasional binge-and-purge episodes, compulsive exercise, returning symptoms of former eating disorders, compulsive overeating, or other food-related behaviors.

Some midlife women with eating problems are carryovers, those who had eating disorders that they were never quite able to shed when they were young. In fact, according to a review completed in 2002, about half of those with anorexia nervosa and at least a third of those with bulimia nervosa carry their eating problems with them into the early and middle stages of adulthood. But many midlife women are developing problematic eating for the first time in their lives. Why? No one really knows for sure. It may be partly because today's midlife woman is more appearance conscious than women of previous generations. Unlike her mother or grandmother, the typical midlife woman today works outside the home. She is competing with younger people every day for jobs, raises, power, and attention and may be loathe to ease into the "plump grandmother" role. Divorce or widowhood may have thrust her back into the singles market, where good looks are the trump card. At the same time, she may be dismayed to find her weight and her waistline steadily increasing, due in part to the hormonal changes of menopause. Fluctuating hormones may also cause changes in her appetite, contribute to blood sugar imbalances, and make her retain water. And statistics show that she is more likely than ever to be seeking help for depression, a condition commonly associated with problem eating. But perhaps the most important force behind her eating problems is the incredibly stressful life she leads.

MIDLIFE IS SYNONYMOUS WITH STRESS

If you're a woman between the ages of 35 and 60, we probably don't have to tell you that you're in what will likely be the most stressful period of your life. At no other time will you have so many responsibilities and experience so many major life changes. In many women, these stressors can trigger problematic eating behaviors. Let's take a closer look at some of the major midlife stress-inducers.

Raising Children

Depending upon when you started your family, your kids may be anywhere from toddlers to teenagers. And though they bring great joy, they also bring heavy responsibilities. Babies and young children need an incredible amount of care and attention. Older children may be more independent, but just coordinating their busy lives and getting them from place to place can be a full-time job, not to mention the sheer work of making sure they get meals, clean clothes, baths, and their homework done without going through a major meltdown. Teenagers bring their own problems and personalities into the mix. Their rebelliousness, increasingly complex lives, and endless interest in pushing it to the edge will, at the very least, test the limits of your tolerance.

No matter what stage your kids are currently in, one thing is certain: They all put unrelenting demands on your time, pocketbook, and patience. Although it's often extremely rewarding, raising kids is undeniably stressful.

Career Challenges

Midlife women also face unique career challenges. If you postponed your career to raise your children (or at least get them into kindergarten), you may find that getting a job now is tougher than you had imagined. Competition is particularly fierce in today's weak labor market, and even brand-new college graduates are having a more difficult time finding a job now than at any time during the past 20 years. The shaky economy and skyrocketing health insurance and pension costs have forced many employers to scale back rather than expand their businesses. They find it's a lot less expensive to increase the workloads of existing employees rather than create additional jobs. In this era of shrinking paychecks, weakening unions, and a smaller labor force, just landing a job can be a major accomplishment. Unfortunately, you'll then be competing with much younger people, fresh out of school, who have the ambition, time, and energy to devote their lives to work.

If you established a career first, then took several years off to start a family, you may discover that your old job is no longer available when you're ready to come back. Or that advances in technology have rendered your job skills obsolete. But even if you've never taken a break and continued to work straight through, once you enter midlife, you may find yourself fending off increasing numbers of young competitors for your job. And if you are a working mom, the special complications that go along with this role—taking extra time off to tend to sick kids, attend school events, or chauffeur the kids to appointments—may make you less attractive to many employers than your younger, unfettered colleagues. Plus, the issues you face as you fight your way up the career ladder can be more difficult to handle as you get older: poor-paying entry-level positions, long hours, ageism, and unfulfilling work.

Whether employed in high-powered careers or minimum-wage jobs, midlife women have one thing in common: We're all faced with the endless and often irreconcilable problem of trying to meet the demands of both job and family. After all, as women we're the major caretakers for our families. If somebody has an emergency, needs to go to the doctor, or has to get picked up at a certain time, who else is he or she going to call? Because we are continually needed, we're constantly torn between our responsibilities at work and those at home.

Empty-Nest Syndrome

After years of doing countless piles of laundry, endlessly preparing meals, and begging your kids to clean their bedrooms, you may think it will be a relief once they finally move out of the house to go to college, start careers, or get married. But for many women, this event can be unexpectedly stressful.

When your grown kids move out, it's normal and natural for you to feel sad, bored, empty, anxious, and lonely—a condition called empty-nest syndrome. This is a major life transition as you move from being the super-responsible, always-needed mom to a woman whose child-rearing responsibilities are, for the most part, finished. Though still a mom, you may start to question your identity as you find yourself with more free time and fewer distractions. The upside is that you'll be free to focus mainly on yourself, your partner, and your own life.

Extended Parenthood

The flip side of empty-nest syndrome is dealing with a nest that doesn't empty soon enough. Back in the 1970s, the average man was married and on his own by age 23; the average woman, by 21. But today's kids are staying home much longer than ever before, either never leaving at all or boomeranging home after college, often living under their parents' roof until they are well into their thirties. In 2000, 12 percent of men and 5 percent of women ages 25 to 34 still lived with at least one parent.

In some cases, kids leave, start an independent life, then come back with grandchildren in tow, wanting to live with you until they get their lives back together. This translates to an extended period of stress, responsibility, and financial strain—not to mention an invasion of your privacy while you put off transitioning into the second half of your life. Some women find that they are never relieved of child-rearing duties. They go straight from raising their own kids to raising their grandchildren. According to the U.S. Census Bureau, in 2002 there were 3.7 million children under the age of 18 living in their grandparents' home. Sixty-five percent of those children had at least one parent also living in the household.

Caring for Aging Parents or Other Relatives

Another problem that's almost completely the province of midlife women is the caretaking of ailing parents. Between the ages of 35 and 44, almost one-fourth of American women become caregivers for their elderly parents, a figure that rises to one-third for those in the 55 to 64 age group. And being a woman makes it highly likely that this demanding new role will fall to you, rather than your brothers (if you have any). Adult daughters are three times more likely to assume the caregiver role than adult sons are, and when it comes to caring for the most-impaired parents, daughters are four times more likely to take up the mantle. Add this to a full- or part-time job (44 to 61 percent of adult daughters who are caregivers are also employed), plus the many other roles you play, and you have a very heavy load to tote.

Although you've always known your parents would age and eventually pass away, when the process actually kicks into gear, it may take you by surprise. After all those years of relying on good ol' Mom and Dad as your backup support system, the roles suddenly reverse and you're taking care of them. This is a difficult adjustment, particularly because your own plate is already filled to overflowing. Right in the middle of dealing with a full-time job, soccer games, ballet lessons, your own hormonal swings, and backed-up plumbing, your mother may be diagnosed with Alzheimer's disease and have to give up driving, or your dad may go on dialysis. You have to take up the slack—accompanying them to doctor's appointments, doing their grocery shopping, taking over their bills, and arranging hospitalization or nursing home stays when necessary. When they finally pass away, you may find yourself awash in both grief and relief, unsure which is greater.

The decline and death of a parent inevitably brings up the issue of your own mortality. Suddenly there is no buffer between you, old age, and death. You are on deck, getting ready to take your place as a member of the older generation. It's a sobering time as you contemplate your own senior years. Are you going to end up with the same physical ailments, the same fading mental abilities, the same problems of old age as your parent had? Though it was once difficult to imagine yourself getting old, all at once it seems much more real.

Financial Burdens

Then there's the problem of how to finance this overloaded, wheezing, bursting-at-the-seams endeavor we call life. Paying bills is not a uniquely midlife phenomenon, but the bulk of society's financial responsibilities lies on our middle-aged shoulders. We bear the brunt of the cost of mortgages, taxes, insurance, day care, cars, lessons, tutoring, furniture, clothes, vacations, college, and weddings.

Although those in midlife have always assumed the greatest financial burden for supporting their families and communities, let's face it: The cost of living is a lot higher today than it was for our parents. Back in the 1950s and 1960s, people easily lived on one income. They had one car, they ate almost all meals at home, Mom may have made many of the clothes, they walked or rode bikes everywhere, and there was no such thing as day care. The total cost of an average home was about the same amount as a schoolteacher made in a year. Even wedding receptions were often backyard buffets that didn't break the budget. Today, the impossibility of living on one income has made it necessary for nearly three-quarters of all mothers with children under 18 to join the labor force, and many of us have already resigned ourselves to the idea of no retirement.

Relationship Troubles

Marital fights, separations, and divorce can happen at any time, of course, but they're particularly frequent during the high-pressure midlife years. Overburdened and overworked, husbands and wives may take each other for granted during these years, spending little time on the relationship because it's the easiest thing to ignore. Careers, children, and endless chores may demand attention right now—but the marriage can often be put on the back burner. Hungry for the love, admiration, or support that they're not getting at home, men and women alike can become vulnerable to infatuations. An exciting new person may appear who seems to fill a void or provide something they're not getting in their marriage. Some marriages give way under the stress; others soldier on. Either way, the midlife years are often a period of crisis within the marriage.

Midlife is also a time for reflection, a time to assess how far we've come and reevaluate where we're going. It could be that the physical changes associated with aging or illness, the death of a parent or a close friend, or the departure of children trigger some intense soul-searching. Some people find themselves asking, "Is that all there is?" They may feel they have topped out in their careers and are trapped in marriages that are no longer fulfilling or satisfying. They may want to escape the old life and start a new one while there is still time, and getting out of the marriage may be the first step. Certain events, such as the youngest child leaving for college, a job ending, or a parent dying, can seem like natural end points for a marriage.

Divorce and Singlehood

Research has shown that there are two high-risk periods for divorce: One spans the first 7 years of the marriage. The second occurs during midlife, when children (if there are any) are young teenagers, a period that some researchers have called the lowest point in marital satisfaction. In the last 30 years, divorce rates have soared, with almost half of first marriages crumbling by the time midlife rolls around. The yearly divorce rate in 2001 was nearly double that seen in 1960, and the proportion of divorced to married individuals has almost quadrupled since 1970, from 47 divorced per 1,000 married in 1970, to 180 per 1,000 in 2001. Clearly, divorce happens, it happens often, and it's not just confined to mismatched newlyweds.

When ranking stressful life events, experts continually put divorce near the top of the list, right under "death of a spouse." And, indeed, divorce can be like a death—the death of a way of life— bringing with it an endless array of stressors: the loss of a loved one, dealing with emotionally wounded children, custody battles, loss of financial status, moving, and adjusting to being single again. Parental pressures increase when a woman finds herself raising her children alone, sharing custody, or fighting with their father over child-rearing methods.

Upping the ante is the prospect of becoming a single person again and venturing into the dating world. The idea of being out there in search of a new partner is frightening for any midlife person. But women have it particularly tough in our current youth-and-beauty-worshipping culture, where they can find themselves competing with women half their age for men who are their contemporaries. Many newly divorced women fall into pathological dieting, excessive exercise, or problem eating behaviors as a reaction to the stress, in an attempt to regain their youthful figures, or for both reasons.

Menopause

It's really unfair that just when we're confronted with mounting family, career, and financial burdens, we also have to face the physical and emotional changes brought about by menopause. Over a period of months or even years, your menstrual periods will become irregular and finally stop completely. As your levels of the hormones estrogen and progesterone fluctuate, the delicate balance that exists between them can be thrown off, triggering anxiety, depression, emotional hypersensitivity, fatigue, hot flashes, migraine headaches, increased sensitivity to pain, and sleeplessness, just to name a few symptoms.

You may also start to worry about losing your sexuality or sexual attractiveness once you're no longer in your reproductive prime. You may wonder if you're less womanly once you've gone through menopause—if men will still find you attractive or if you're losing an important part of your identity. Menopause can bring about changes in the way you look, feel, and respond physically and emotionally. Luckily, by paying attention to your eating and exercise habits, and seeing your doctor regularly, you can do much to ease menopausal symptoms and stay comfortable and confident.

Aging

As you ease into your middle years, it's inevitable that you will notice certain physical signs of aging. Your overall strength declines somewhat, and your muscles can get strained and sprained more easily as they become weaker and less resilient (especially if you don't exercise regularly). You may gain weight more easily and find it harder to lose those extra pounds because of the age-related slowing of your metabolism. In fact, researchers at the University of Pittsburgh, studying 485 premenopausal women ages 42 to 50, found that the women's weight increased an average of 5 pounds over a 3-year period, with 20 percent of the group showing a weight gain of 10 or more pounds. Eight years after menopause, the average woman weighed 12 pounds more than she did at the start of the study.

Yet due to a redistribution of fatty tissue, the fat in your face seems to disappear with no effort at all, leaving sagging skin and increased wrinkles in its wake. Your abdominal muscles become softer, your breasts start to lose firmness, your skin and hair may thin and dry out, and age spots can appear on the areas of your body that have seen the most sun. As women who live in a culture that worships beauty and youth, most of us find these changes unsettling, at the very least. But for some, they are devastating.

Women whose identities depend upon their looks (such as actresses and models) can be thrown into a panic by age-related changes. But even the woman down the street, whose livelihood isn't related to her looks, can experience anxiety or a sense of mourning as her youthful face and body begin to show signs of aging.

WHAT IS ALL THIS STRESS DOING TO US?

The combination of career challenges, empty-nest syndrome, increasing family responsibilities, marital problems, menopause, and all the rest adds up to an extremely stressful period in any woman's life. So what does that mean in terms of your health? We can sum it up in one sentence: Stress wreaks havoc on just about all of the major body systems and can cause major diseases and difficulties—both physical and psychological.

Stress sets off the equivalent of a four-stage fire alarm in your body. Your adrenal glands send out a flood of chemicals (stress hormones) that instantly raise your blood pressure and speed up your heart rate, breathing rate, and metabolism. They also stimulate the breakdown of muscle and visceral protein to provide a ready source of amino acids for the repair of tissue damage. And they mobilize fatty tissue for extra fuel so that your body will have the energy and power to run a mile or fight to the death, if necessary. As your blood supply is diverted to your larger muscles, your hands and feet get cold and clammy, and the sandwich you had for lunch lies like a lump in your stomach. Your pupils dilate, and your diaphragm locks. You're ready for whatever comes your way.

This is all great if you happen to be attacked by a wild animal, but if you're simply in the middle of an argument with your husband or just trying to rush to the school to pick up the kids on time, this shower of stress hormones is overkill. And if you're under chronic stress (the typical state for most midlife women), constant exposure to this high-powered chemical brew will make you much more likely to suffer from certain serious physical problems, including heart disease, cancer, chronic fatigue, arthritis, asthma, migraines, obesity, accelerated aging, ulcerative colitis, chronic pain, and diabetes.

Stress is just as destructive on the psychological front, with symptoms including depression, anxiety, a feeling of powerlessness, hostility, anger, irritability, resentment, apathy, impatience, obsessions, fears, and phobias. In other words, chronic stress can make you feel terrible. Depression and anxiety, in particular, are two hallmarks of midlife for many women and are greatly exacerbated by perimenopause and menopause, work overload, and other midlife stressors.

In short, stress makes us feel like hell—physically and psychologically. We yearn to feel better, to escape the nonstop stress and frustration. So when things get to be too much to bear, it's not surprising that many of us fall into unhealthy behaviors. We may become workaholics; we may drink too much alcohol or get hooked on prescription or over-the-counter drugs. But much more often, we turn to food.

FOOD: THE "ACCEPTABLE" VICE

Food is a source of pleasure, comfort, amusement, sedation, and distraction, making it a highly attractive commodity. And we're surrounded by it—at home, at work, at social occasions, at the movie theater, in the shopping mall, at the baseball stadium. There's even a cable network devoted to it. It seems to be everywhere. In fact, you may be hard-pressed to think of a situation that doesn't involve food. And, whether we like it or not, as women, we're intimately involved with it. We can spend an inordinate amount of time planning meals, grocery shopping, cooking, freezing, packaging, preparing, and serving food to our families and friends.

Food is perhaps the most easily available, socially acceptable, hard-to-resist substance in existence that can help us escape from

"STRESSED-OUT" EATING HABITS

When you're feeling stressed, you might be tempted to skip a meal or resort to eating convenience foods instead of taking the time to cook dinner. And when your energy starts to lag, coffee or cola might seem like just the thing you need to keep yourself going. Yet by resorting to poor eating habits such as these, you may unwittingly be increasing your stress levels. Consider the following eating habits and the negative consequences of each.

Skipping meals. When you don't eat regularly, your blood sugar can drop, increasing physical and psychological stress as you experience hunger, weakness, irritability, moodiness, and fatigue.

Bingeing. Eating unusually large amounts of food overloads the digestive system and can leave you feeling bloated, nauseated, and exhausted. But the psychological effects—depression, anxiety, intense fear of weight gain, self-loathing, and hopelessness—may be even more difficult to bear.

Eating lots of convenience foods. Typically high in saturated fat, sodium, and preservatives while low in nutrients and fiber, convenience foods can fill you up but leave you in a state of under-nutrition. Over time, eating too many of these foods can lead to nutrient imbalances that can inter-

the stress of our lives—even if only for a few moments. No wonder food is such a tantalizing trap for some people.

How can food be misused? We might eat too much, or too little. We might eat too much of a certain kind of food, especially to the exclusion of nutritious foods. But generally, we misuse food by using it to compensate for some imbalance in life.

If a person is abusing alcohol or drugs, it's easy to spot the aberrant behavior. But it's a lot less obvious with food. After all, everybody eats, so no one's going to think twice if they see you eating. On the other hand, it also seems as if just about everybody

fere with your overall health and your psychological state. Irritability, lethargy, headaches, low blood sugar, fatigue, anxiety, and depression may be at least partially due to poor nutrition habits.

Eating sugary foods. When eaten by themselves, foods high in sugar or refined carbohydrates (like white bread, white rice, instant potatoes, or cornflakes) make your blood sugar rise. The hormone insulin then clears the sugar from the bloodstream but can overdo it, leaving you tired, shaky, hungry, irritable, and moody. Flooding your system with insulin is hard on your body and over time can contribute to water retention, diabetes, heart disease, high cholesterol, hormone imbalance, and obesity.

Increasing caffeine intake. Caffeine stimulates the release of the hormone adrenaline, which not only makes you more alert but also more irritable and anxious. Caffeine intake can also contribute to mood swings, insomnia, and the depletion of B vitamins (which are important to glucose metabolism), and it may play a role in recurring depression.

Increasing alcohol intake. Alcohol, which itself is a depressant, increases the likelihood of depression even more and can intensify feelings of fatigue, hopelessness, anxiety, and despair.

---

is on a diet. So if you're picking at a green salad and sipping iced tea for lunch, no one's going to worry that you're restricting your food intake abnormally. In fact, you'll probably be applauded for it. Yet as normal as the acts of eating or dieting may appear to be, either can stray into unhealthy food behaviors—Runaway Eating—under certain conditions. And Runaway Eating can be just as habit forming as alcohol or drugs.

At the very least, Runaway Eating can have a profoundly negative impact on your self-image, relationships, professional performance, and quality of life. In its most severe forms, the dire consequences of disordered eating can include osteoporosis, heart problems, kidney dysfunction, anemia, changes in brain structure, gastrointestinal problems, and, sometimes, even death.

WHY CAN'T WE STOP OURSELVES?

A century ago, women's relationship with food was markedly different from what it is today. Preparing food was a creative and sensual task that gave most women great satisfaction. The serving of meals to their families, the gifts of homemade foods to the sick, the special foods painstakingly prepared for holidays and important events were all ways that women could nurture their families, express love, and occupy an important role in the family unit. Food was a part of family cohesiveness; family members were nurtured psychologically as well as physically at mealtimes. Women sat down with their families, connected with their loved ones, ate until they felt satisfied, and stopped when they'd had enough. Food wasn't an issue in those days (except for those who weren't getting enough of it). An ample female body was normal, natural, comfortable, and expected.

But for many of us today, food has become the enemy. It tempts us, makes us fat, and causes us to feel bad about ourselves. Food is something we want to avoid (as much as possible), ignore, control, and defeat. Too much food, we believe, can result in social rejection and a lack of power, love, or sex. For many of us, cooking isn't considered pleasurable or an expression of love anymore—it's drudgery. We'd much rather go out, grab some fast food, or throw something in the microwave. Through endless dieting, we've learned to override our bodies' natural signals telling us it's time to eat or time to stop eating. Instead, we make those decisions with our minds—minds that tell us we have to stop short of satisfying ourselves or continue to gorge long after our stomachs are full. We've become disconnected from food and from our own bodies.

Yet our bodies and minds continue to be hungry for physical and psychological nourishment. Our dieting; poor nutrition habits; excessive consumption of processed foods, fast foods, sugar, salt, and food additives; and lack of real, fresh, highly nutritious foods have left us with appetites that are never satisfied. And our fast-paced, high-stress, competitive, impersonal lives have left us feeling underloved, underappreciated, and undernourished psychologically. Sometimes we may think that the answer to our hunger is to stuff down a quart of ice cream or a dozen doughnuts, but it never is. Or it may seem that we can win the war with food by dieting like crazy or exercising for hours a day. But we can never win this way. Only when we learn to make friends with food, reconnect with our bodies, and heed the natural calls of both body and mind will we find peace. In this book, we will give you the tools you need to make peace with food; learn to love, respect, and listen to your body; and finally find relief from Runaway Eating.

CHAPTER 2

What Is Runaway Eating?

S onia is a 57-year-old flight attendant who went on a crash diet when her second husband ran off with her daughter's best friend. Feeling unattractive, spurned, and over-the-hill, she decided she had to do something about her slightly plump figure if she was ever going to find another romance. "I'm out in the singles market again," she says gloomily, "and that means I've got to have something to sell."

During a 3-month period, Sonia followed a strict diet that left her thinner than she'd ever been in her adult life. At 5 feet 2, she now weighs about 100 pounds, down 35 pounds from her starting weight. Though the tiny portions she allows herself usually leave her still feeling hungry, she is scared to death to stop dieting for fear she'll gain back all the weight she lost.

Sonia doesn't fit the description of a person with anorexia nervosa, because her weight isn't low enough. But her eating behaviors and attitudes are far from healthy.

<hr />

As vice president of advertising for a major movie studio, 38-year-old Catherine is in charge of a top-notch creative team that has helped catapult the studio's last three pictures to number one at the box office. Her underlings love her, praising her for her great communication skills, fearless leadership, and savvy promotional instincts. Catherine's personal life is also enviable: She is married to a successful movie director and has twin 2-year-old boys and a huge house in the Hollywood Hills. To top it all off, she bears a striking resemblance to Meg Ryan.

But some nights, when Catherine finally drags herself home from work, exhausted yet keyed up, she heads straight for the kitchen and starts eating like there's no tomorrow. One of her favorite splurges is peanut butter and honey on bread (sometimes as many as five slices) accompanied by a couple of glasses of milk. Her husband usually picks up some take-out food on his way home, so once the boys are asleep, they have a quick dinner in front of the TV. Then, about 10:00 P.M., Catherine starts craving rocky road ice cream. Before she knows it, she's eaten an entire pint all by herself. And on some nights, she goes back for more. As her clothes get tighter and her figure gets rounder, she knows she needs to get a handle on her eating. But somehow, worrying about her weight and thinking about diets just make her want to eat more.

"This is terrible," she keeps telling herself. "I'm in control of everything but myself."

Catherine doesn't fit the profile of someone with binge-eating disorder because she doesn't binge often enough. Some nights she overdoes it, but other nights she eats normally. Yet these occasional binges are certainly unhealthy eating behaviors.

Forty-five-year-old Toni is an administrative assistant at a large accounting firm. She never seems to eat much at work; she's not a snacker, and her lunch usually consists of a salad and a diet soft drink. But when she gets home, she feels she can let down her guard and eat. After all, she's been "good" all day. Dinner is usually substantial, but once her husband retires to the study and she settles down to watch television, the fun really begins. Out come the M&Ms, the ice cream, and (her personal favorite) the potato chips. Toni can eat an entire bag of chips (sometimes two) in one sitting—and often, she does just that.

But at a certain point, she realizes that she's gone too far. All those calories! She knows she's going to pack on the pounds if she continues. So sometimes she closets herself in the bathroom and forces herself to vomit. Afterward, feeling sick, tired, and disgusted with herself, she always makes a solemn vow to follow a strict diet the next day and get control of herself.

Toni's condition doesn't meet the rigid criteria for bulimia nervosa, because she binges and purges only about once a week. Still, her eating is clearly out of control.

THE RUNAWAY EATER: FLYING UNDER THE RADAR

There is no doubt that Catherine, Sonia, and Toni—along with millions of other women—show signs of disturbed eating behavior. This behavior leaves them feeling out of control and, if not addressed, can damage their physical, mental, and emotional health. Yet because their symptoms don't meet all the criteria necessary to be diagnosed as an official eating disorder, their problems often go unrecognized and untreated.

What most of us don't realize is that eating problems exist on a continuum. You don't just wake up one day with a full-blown eating disorder. Disordered eating is a gradual process that includes a whole gamut of behaviors, ranging from something as benign as weight preoccupation or an occasional lapse into compulsive overeating, to the recognized eating disorders of bulimia nervosa, anorexia nervosa, and binge-eating disorder. Although the thoughts, feelings, and behaviors associated with problematic eating may be mild initially, they can gradually worsen until they become overwhelming. Unfortunately, most people don't seek help (or even believe they have a problem) until their eating troubles become severe.

Thus, women like Catherine, Sonia, and Toni slip through the diagnostic and treatment cracks and may go for years thinking that they're just undisciplined, lazy, or somehow flawed because they can't seem to control their weight, shape, or eating-related behaviors. But these behaviors may *not* be due to simple character deficits or bad habits: They may be the result of a complex web of personality, familial, biological, and sociocultural factors. Thousands of women who feel bad physically or emotionally, or who are cracking under life's stresses and strains, find themselves turning to food, dieting, purging, or excessive exercise for relief. We have labeled such behaviors Runaway Eating, a name with a double meaning: *Their eating-related behaviors have run away with them* and *they are eating to run away from other problems.*

WHAT CONSTITUTES RUNAWAY EATING?

There are probably very few of us who, at some point, haven't overindulged in a huge bowl of ice cream or polished off an entire bag of chips. But Runaway Eating is not just about eating to excess. It's about using food or food-related activities as a way to deal with your problems, and it can include other emotion-driven food behaviors, such as strict dieting, excessive exercise, and overuse of laxatives or diuretics. These behaviors can be fueled by depression, anxiety, low self-esteem, an intense need for control, and an overwhelming desire for acceptance, among other things. In effect, these eating behaviors serve as a way to run away from emotional problems. As a rule of thumb, if you consistently use food or food-related behaviors to deal with unpleasant feelings *and* you feel that these behaviors are out of control, you've entered into the territory of Runaway Eating.

Eating to Deal with Your Feelings

Practically all of us eat for emotional reasons some of the time, but when eating-related behaviors become your primary way of dealing with your feelings, you've become a Runaway Eater. Some women eat to excess when they're angry, depressed, or anxious; others may purge or simply stop eating at these times. Some overeat to reward or soothe themselves or ease boredom or fatigue. Others exercise excessively or purge to rid themselves of guilt, anger, or shame. Some use food, dieting, or purging to distract themselves, procrastinate, or simply to blot out the world for a while. What all of these behaviors have in common is the "stuffing down" of unhappy feelings.

Instead of getting the problem out in the open and dealing with it in a constructive way, a Runaway Eater will internalize the problem so that she can hide it or ignore it. Ironically, although she thinks she is ridding herself of the problem by running away, stuffing down her emotions only makes everything worse. Eventually, this becomes such a standard way of operating that she's not even aware she's doing it.

Feeling out of Control around Food

When you feel powerless to stop your unhealthy food-related behaviors (whether you're overeating, binge-eating, purging, dieting, exercising excessively, or anything else) even though you know they're hurting you, you have become a Runaway Eater. Try as you may, you keep coming back to the old habits, automatic reactions, and hurtful ways of dealing with your body and your world.

Although Runaway Eating is rooted in the same psychological and sociocultural factors that cause the clinically defined eating disorders, the symptoms and results aren't as extreme. For example, the Runaway Eater doesn't starve herself down to a dangerously low weight, but she does have some of the same pathological attitudes toward food, weight, and dieting seen in someone with anorexia nervosa. The Runaway Eater may not binge on huge quantities of food and then make herself vomit, but like those with bulimia nervosa, she may overeat to ease tension and depression, feeling powerless to stop herself.

You may be suffering from Runaway Eating if you do any of the following:

- Feel as though your eating or weight-control strategies have spiraled out of control
- Bounce from strict dieting to eating everything in sight
- Exercise like crazy to keep the weight off and are afraid to stop
- Binge-eat for emotional reasons like boredom, anxiety, depression, or frustration

- Induce vomiting once in a while if you feel you've eaten too much
- Sometimes try to speed food through your body by using laxatives, diuretics, or enemas
- Induce vomiting or use laxatives, diuretics, or enemas even if you haven't binged
- Chew and spit out your food to avoid taking in calories

HOW MANY PEOPLE HAVE RUNAWAY EATING?

It's impossible to pin down exactly how many people are suffering from Runaway Eating because most have probably never even imagined that they might have a mild form of an eating disorder. Dawn, a 54-year-old elementary school teacher, reacted to this idea in a typical fashion: "Eating disorder? I don't starve, and I don't throw up, so I certainly don't have one of those!"

Between 3 and 5 percent of the population has been diagnosed with a clinically defined eating disorder, but it's estimated that up to 10 percent may have milder forms of eating disorders and that another 10 to 15 percent may experience isolated symptoms, like occasional binge-eating, that leave them feeling out of control. This means that some 25 percent of the female population may be living with an undiagnosed, untreated condition that hurts both their psychological and physical health.

Sometimes Runaway Eating can morph into a bona fide eating disorder, sometimes it may simply stay at a low level, and sometimes it may disappear on its own. But no matter how mild or infrequent the bouts of Runaway Eating may be, they indicate that eating-related behaviors have become a harmful way of dealing with other problems, and they warn that a clinically defined eating disorder may be on the horizon.

WHAT FORMS CAN RUNAWAY EATING TAKE?

Although all Runaway Eaters use food or food-related behaviors to deal with problems that have nothing to do with food, there are three general types of Runaway Eaters.

- The Restricting Runaway Eater
- The Bingeing Runaway Eater
- The Bingeing/Compensating Runaway Eater

Many Runaway Eaters fall into a single category, but some may move from one type to another over time or even engage in all three kinds of behavior. Although these three types may appear to be quite different from each other on the surface, the driving forces behind them are remarkably similar, including low self-esteem, mood fluctuations, depression, the belief that being thin will solve most problems, and the use of food to deal with unpleasant emotions.

The Restricting Runaway Eater

The Restricting Runaway Eater shows many of the same symptoms seen in a person with anorexia nervosa (AN) but in a milder form. Both are terrified of gaining weight or being fat. This allows them to override their hunger signals and cut back food to dangerously low levels, sometimes even to the point of starvation.

Some ignore their body signals for so long that they eventually stop feeling hungry altogether, but most Restricting Runaway Eaters have a strong desire to eat and may spend almost every waking moment thinking about food. The only thing that is more interesting to them than food is being thin and in control. This

YOU COULD BE A RESTRICTING RUNAWAY EATER IF . . .

- You want to maintain a body weight that is below normal for your height and frame.
- You are constantly on a diet.
- You have an intense fear of gaining weight or getting fat. This fear doesn't go away, no matter how much weight you lose.
- You feel "fat" even when you are of normal or below-normal weight for your height and frame.
- You place a great deal of importance on your body weight or shape when you evaluate yourself.
- You believe that you can't be happy or successful until you reach a certain weight.

type of Runaway Eater checks the mirror several times a day; tries on and often buys clothes that are too small, hoping to fit into them; and feels certain that happiness will elude her until she reaches a certain weight.

The main difference between the Restricting Runaway Eater and the woman with anorexia nervosa is weight. The woman with anorexia gets her weight down to a dangerously low level for her height (usually less than 85 percent of her ideal body weight), and the Restricting Runaway Eater hovers just around the low end of normal. It could be just a matter of time, however, before her weight drops to anorexic levels. Also, the Restricting Runaway Eater may not restrict her food as much or as consistently as does the woman with anorexia. She may go through periods of relatively normal eating, and when she does restrict, it may not be to the starvation level. But the fixation on food and the fear of weight gain are ever-present companions.

What's the Difference between Being a Restricting Runaway Eater and Being Very Thin?

How do you know if you're a Restricting Runaway Eater or just very thin? First of all, the naturally thin person doesn't think too much about food except at mealtime. When she eats, she does so until her body signals her to stop, then she goes about her business. But a Restricting Runaway Eater is obsessed with food, weight, and shape. Her self-esteem is very much dependent on her ability to get thin, stay thin, and fit into smaller-and-smaller-size clothes. To her, losing weight means self-control and achievement; gaining weight means failure and shame.

The Restricting Runaway Eater has a distorted sense of her own body size and shape and feels "fat" no matter how thin she gets. She is compulsive about dieting and losing weight and may weigh herself many times a day, measure certain areas of her body over and over, and touch her body to see if her bones are protruding far enough.

What Restricting Runaway Eating Can Do to Your Body

When you restrict your food intake, your vital functions may slow to conserve energy: Your body will begin to burn calories at a lower rate, your heart rate slows, your blood pressure may drop, and your circulation may become sluggish and poor. As a result, you might feel light-headed, dizzy, and cold no matter what the weather is. Also, Restricting Runaway Eating can progress to full-blown anorexia nervosa, bringing with it all of the associated health risks.

If your level of body fat drops too low, you may lose your menstrual periods (if you are premenopausal), because some estrogen is produced from fatty tissue. This decreases your chances of conceiving a baby. It's as if the body realizes that the food supply is too low to support a pregnancy. The risk of miscarriage, premature birth, and birth defects increases in women with eating disorders. And even those who are at a normal weight but have a history of an eating disorder have an increased risk of having a cesarean section, premature delivery, and low-birth-weight baby. Also, because estrogen is necessary for bone health, a low level of body fat can contribute to the development of osteoporosis.

More-extreme effects of eating too little over a long period of time include anemia, electrolyte imbalances, impaired immune response, disturbed pancreatic function, kidney failure, arrhythmias, heart failure, and even death.

What Restricting Runaway Eating Can Do to Your Mind and Emotions

When you're deprived of sufficient food, you can become withdrawn, depressed, and irritable. You think constantly about food and eating. You may have trouble sleeping and become so obsessed with food that you even dream about it. When you finally do eat, you might observe certain rituals like chewing each bite a certain number of times, cutting up all of your food into very tiny pieces, or mixing everything together on your plate. You might also hide food away (but never eat it) or cook big, elaborate meals for others just to be near food, but never tasting it yourself.

Like those with anorexia, Restricting Runaway Eaters may suffer from anxiety, obsessive-compulsive traits, perfectionism, low self-esteem, and hopelessness. No one knows whether these feelings are the cause or the result of restrictive eating, but it seems clear that each feeds the other. The negative feelings increase the food restriction, and the food restriction increases the negative feelings.

The Restricting Runaway Eater may also find that her food and weight obsessions take a toll on her relationships. She may refuse social engagements that include food (and that's practically all of them!) and lie to those close to her about what she has or hasn't eaten. Her intense focus on weight and food can also turn off partners (or prospective partners) who get tired of constantly being asked, "Do I look fat?"

The Bingeing Runaway Eater

The Bingeing Runaway Eater binges, or eats to excess, primarily to make herself feel better. A binge can involve a huge amount of food (in some cases as many as 20,000 calories) or a much smaller amount (say, two pieces of cake). Binge foods are usually those that are high in sugar and fat and easy to eat in large quantities, like ice cream, cake, cookies, peanut butter, jam, honey, or candy.

Eating may be pleasurable at the beginning of a binge, but as more food is eaten, the enjoyment turns to revulsion and disgust at what's taking place. Usually, the food is eaten very rapidly, barely chewed, and may be washed down with plenty of liquid. Agitation, tension, and guilt may accompany the binge, wiping out any satisfaction that eating might normally bring. Sometimes those who binge feel as if they're in an altered state of consciousness, barely aware of what they're doing. There is a sense that the binge is inevitable and that they are powerless to stop it. Embarrassment, shame, and disgust lead most people to binge in secret, safe from the criticism of others. However, Bingeing Runaway Eaters don't purge, diet restrictively, or exercise excessively to try to get rid of the excess calories. They binge and leave it at that.

Binge-eating is much more common than either anorexia or bulimia. It is estimated to affect between 2 and 5 percent of the

YOU COULD BE A BINGEING RUNAWAY EATER IF . . .

- You eat unusually large amounts of food in a short period of time.
- During these episodes, you feel unable to control your eating.
- You eat at a much faster pace than normal during these episodes.
- You eat until you're uncomfortably full during these episodes.
- After these episodes, you feel disgusted, depressed, or very guilty.
- You eat alone because you're embarrassed about how much you eat.
- You don't fast, diet stringently, purge, or exercise excessively to compensate for these episodes.
- You have recurring episodes of this kind of eating.

U.S. population and up to half of those in self-help or commercial weight-loss programs. Although not yet officially recognized as an eating disorder, there is a name for more-severe, recurring episodes of binge-eating: binge-eating disorder (BED).

What's the Difference between Bingeing Runaway Eating, Overeating, and Binge-Eating Disorder?

Overeating is simply eating more than your body needs to maintain good health and a normal body weight for your frame. Bingeing Runaway Eating involves eating a larger-than-usual amount of food within a short period of time while feeling that your eating is out of control. Some Runaway Eaters find that they can't stop themselves until they are physically unable to continue eating, are interrupted, become exhausted, or run out of food. The out-of-control feeling is absent in simple overeating.

The main difference between Bingeing Runaway Eating and binge-eating disorder lies in the frequency or duration of the bingeing. Those with BED binge an average of at least 2 days a week for at least 6 months. Those with Bingeing Runaway Eating may binge only occasionally or for shorter periods of time. But it's important to remember that there is no firm dividing line. These behaviors lie on a continuum and are unhealthy, no matter how seldom they happen.

What Bingeing Runaway Eating Can Do to Your Body

Eating until you are very full can make you feel bloated, nauseated, or unable to breathe well because of a distended stomach pressing on your diaphragm. By far, the most common "side effect" of binge-eating is weight gain. Though not all binge-eaters are obese or overweight, and not all of those who are overweight are binge-eaters, bingeing can maintain any existing weight problem and in some cases make it worse.

What Bingeing Runaway Eating Can Do to Your Mind and Emotions

If you are a Bingeing Runaway Eater, you may find yourself suffering from depression, anxiety, guilt, self-loathing, or shame. You don't want to talk about your problems or your eating behaviors, so you isolate yourself from others, although love, friendship, and caring are the things that you need most. You may hurry home from social engagements so that you can have a date with the pantry. You may even wish that your partner or family members would leave the house so that you can be alone with food.

When you're focused on food, diets, eating, or weight issues, you tend to concentrate less on family, friends, hobbies, work, and many of the other things that make life worth living. A wall of secrecy descends between you and your loved ones. Intimacy decreases, your mood suffers, and your joy in life plummets.

The Bingeing/Compensating Runaway Eater

As the name suggests, this type of Runaway Eating involves a two-step process: bingeing on large amounts of food eaten in a short period of time, then compensating for the extra calories by purging, fasting, or engaging in excessive exercise. Because this type of Runaway Eater gets rid of some of the calorie load, she keeps her weight at an average to slightly above-average level.

Like her restricting counterpart, this type of Runaway Eater is intensely afraid of getting fat, because her self-esteem is very dependent upon her shape and weight. But because she's more impulsive than the restricting type, sticking to a diet for any length of time can be impossible for her. She may try hard, but eventually she'll abandon her diet and end up eating large quantities of food to relieve the stress.

Once she's eaten all of that food, though, the Bingeing/Compensating Runaway Eater finds herself engulfed in a wave of panic, fear, and guilt, believing she must do something to get rid of it before it turns to fat. She may do one or more of the following:

- Put herself on a very restrictive diet
- Fast or simply starve herself
- Purge by inducing vomiting to get the food out of her system
- Abuse laxatives, diuretics, or enemas, or use other unhealthy methods to try to rid her body of the food
- Exercise excessively to try to burn off those extra calories

This category of Runaway Eaters also includes those who simply purge, without bingeing first.

YOU COULD BE A BINGEING/COMPENSATING RUNAWAY EATER IF . . .

- Your self-worth depends on your body shape and weight.
- You have recurring or occasional episodes of binge-eating.
- You feel out of control while eating.
- You have recurring episodes of compensatory behavior to avoid weight gain, such as dieting, fasting, vomiting, exercising excessively, or abusing laxatives, diuretics, or enemas.

What's the Difference between Bingeing/Compensating Runaway Eating and Bulimia Nervosa?

Both this type of Runaway Eating and bulimia nervosa involve repeated binge-eating episodes plus the compensatory behaviors. Both include a deep dissatisfaction with body shape and weight and a desperate desire to regain control. The difference between the two lies in their frequency or duration. A person with bulimia binge-eats and compensates for the binge an average of at least twice a week for at least 3 months. The Bingeing/Compensating Runaway Eater may binge-eat and use compensatory behaviors less often, only occasionally, or over a shorter period of time.

How Does Purging Affect Weight?

Most of the methods used by Bingeing/Compensating Runaway Eaters to rid themselves of the food—and calories—that they took in during a binge are, at best, ineffective. Fasting, starving, or restrictive dieting slows the metabolism and makes it even more difficult to burn off calories. Self-induced vomiting doesn't usually empty the stomach completely, and a good portion of what was eaten has already moved or will quickly move into the intestines.

Laxatives and enemas work only in the large intestine or rectum, after most of the calories have already been absorbed. And diuretics simply rid the body of water and electrolytes; they don't affect the fat stores. For these reasons, most Bingeing/Compensating Runaway Eaters are not excessively thin; they tend to be of average or slightly above-average weight.

What's the Definition of Excessive Exercise?

Excessive exercise is considered a compensatory behavior, but how do you know if you're doing too much? The answer is simple: If you're exercising for more than 1 hour a day every day *for the sole purpose of avoiding weight gain,* or if you beat yourself up emotionally for missing a day, or if you continue to exercise even though you are injured or exhausted, you're engaging in excessive exercise. This is very common behavior for those with the clinically defined eating disorders of anorexia or bulimia nervosa: As much as 75 percent of either group uses exercise to ward off weight gain. Although most excessive exercisers will insist that they have to lose weight in order to look good or stay in shape, their underlying issues are control, power, and self-esteem.

To find out if you are exercising excessively, ask yourself:

- Do you exercise more often and more intensely than necessary to maintain good health?
- Does the thought of missing a day of exercise make you anxious?
- Do you define yourself according to your athletic performance?
- Are you always dissatisfied with your athletic performance?
- Do you find yourself constantly thinking about dieting and weight loss?

- Do you exercise even when you're injured?
- Do you beat yourself up emotionally when you miss a workout?
- Does your family, work, or personal life suffer as you devote more and more time to exercise?
- Do you spend more than an hour a day every day exercising for the sole purpose of controlling your weight?

If you answered yes to any of these, you may be exercising too much.

What Bingeing/Compensating Runaway Eating Can Do to Your Body

Bingeing repeatedly can stretch the stomach beyond normal capacity, but purging and the other compensatory actions are the more dangerous behaviors. Vomiting can irritate or rupture the esophagus and cause aspiration pneumonia if the vomit is inhaled. Continual exposure to stomach acid erodes tooth enamel, making the teeth look ragged and increasing dental cavities. It's not unusual for those who induce vomiting to spend thousands of dollars on cosmetic dentistry. Self-induced vomiting can also cause dehydration, electrolyte imbalances, chronic kidney problems, broken blood vessels in the eyes or face, vitamin and mineral deficiencies, swollen parotid glands (which give the face a "chipmunk cheek" appearance), and abrasions on the knuckles. Drugs used to induce vomiting can be toxic to the heart and, when used repeatedly, can lead to heart dysfunction or heart failure.

Compensating for a binge by using laxatives or diuretics is also dangerous. Prolonged use of laxatives can make it practically impossible to have normal bowel movements and can cause serious gastrointestinal problems. Repeated use of diuretics can deplete your stores of potassium, which may cause an irregular heartbeat, fatigue, weakness, or other problems.

And even exercise, when used as a compensatory tool, can be detrimental to your health by causing dehydration, stress fractures, increased risk of injury, degenerative arthritis, or premature loss of the menstrual cycle.

What Bingeing/Compensating Runaway Eating Can Do to Your Mind and Emotions

If you have this type of Runaway Eating, you may feel panicked after a binge and then experience some relief after engaging in a compensatory action. But you are probably also well aware that these behaviors are destructive and abnormal, and you may feel disgusted and ashamed of yourself. Depression, irritability, headaches, exhaustion, and guilt are direct results of the binge/compensate cycle. These feelings exacerbate the low self-esteem, worry, and out-of-control feelings that started the whole process, making you feel worse than when you began and more desperate to lose weight.

Because bingeing and the compensatory behaviors are usually done in secret, the isolation, denial, lying, and breach of trust can damage key relationships. Your food and weight obsessions may keep you from focusing on the important people in your life or handling your responsibilities effectively. Your loved ones may find your behavior impossible to understand, widening the gap between you and them, and making your relationships more difficult.

WHAT ARE THE WARNING SIGNS OF RUNAWAY EATING?

Eating problems exist on a continuum, so Runaway Eating can also show up in lesser degrees than those spelled out above. If any of the following describes your behaviors, you may have eating-related trouble on the horizon.

- Constant dieting
- Repeated weight fluctuations
- Often thinking about food or diets
- Feeling guilty about eating
- Occasional lapses into out-of-control eating
- "Grazing" all day instead of eating regular meals
- Dividing food into clear-cut categories of "good" and "bad"
- Avoiding certain activities or people because they're associated with food
- Feeling depressed, anxious, or worthless because your weight is "all wrong"
- Believing that weight loss is the answer to most or all of your problems

Healthy eating, on the other hand, means eating when you're hungry and stopping when you're not. It means knowing the difference between physical hunger and emotional hunger and distinguishing between being satiated and being stuffed. If you're eating any other way, you may be a Runaway Eater.

To better evaluate whether you are a Runaway Eater—or are on the verge of developing an eating problem—work through the quiz on page 44.

YOU CAN LET GO OF RUNAWAY EATING

Until now, if you suffered from Runaway Eating, you were pretty much on your own. Although psychologists have used sophisticated methods to identify and treat clinically defined eating disorders for more than 30 years, if you were flying under the radar by not exhibiting the severe symptoms of a serious eating disorder, you probably didn't seek or receive any kind of help. At best, you may have joined a diet club. Or your doctor may have given you a standard diet, plus instructions to exercise more. Yet these well-meaning "treatments" probably just made your problem worse.

We now know that eating disorders don't just suddenly pop up out of nowhere. They exist on a continuum that ranges from something as benign as weight preoccupation or an occasional lapse into compulsive overeating, to the recognized eating disorders of bulimia nervosa, anorexia nervosa, and binge-eating disorder. The common denominator is that all of these symptoms, from mild to severe, stem from the same cluster of biological, psychological and sociocultural origins. And that means that the same basic techniques psychologists and dietitians use to treat the clinically defined eating disorders will work just as well for Runaway Eating. It is the basis of this book: We offer to those who have milder (but still troubling) problems the same basic psychological and nutritional therapies that work for those with full-blown eating disorders.

Now, at last, there's a way to get a handle on your out-of-control eating behavior. By following our 8-point self-treatment plan, you'll find ways to ferret out the underlying problems that cause your eating trouble and that keep it in motion. You'll learn how to address these problems, handle new ones as they come up, and prevent future complications, all without falling back into the old destructive eating behavior. If you're tired of being controlled by food and eating, this program is for you.

But before delving into the 8-point plan, let's take a brief look at what causes Runaway Eating, what keeps it going, and who's most likely to develop it.

ARE YOU A RUNAWAY EATER?

The following quiz is specially designed to help you determine whether or not Runaway Eating is a problem for you. It also measures the severity of your symptoms. To complete it, answer "true" or "false" for each of the following statements.

__ 1. Your weight has dropped to an abnormally low point or risen to an abnormally high point.

__ 2. You make excuses for not eating while others are having a meal.

__ 3. You divide foods or behaviors into clear-cut "good" or "bad" categories.

__ 4. You eat a lot of noncalorie foods such as diet soft drinks, coffee, mustard, gum, or spices to satisfy your appetite.

__ 5. You often use food to reward yourself.

__ 6. You are defensive about your weight.

__ 7. You panic when you can't weigh yourself.

__ 8. Eating makes you feel guilty.

__ 9. Your weight seems to go up and down, with dramatic fluctuations of 10 pounds or more.

__ 10. You are extremely concerned about your appearance, which is the defining feature of your self-esteem.

__ 11. You always seem to be on a diet.

__ 12. You worry about your body not being small enough, thin enough, or good enough.

__ 13. You compare yourself physically with others and feel inferior.

__ 14. You touch certain parts of your body (such as your stomach, thighs, or hips) several times a day to make sure they feel thin enough.

__ 15. You feel in control when you're at a weight that is abnormally low for you.

___ 16. You often eat when you're not hungry.

___ 17. You completely avoid certain foods like sugar or bread because they are "fattening."

___ 18. You can't get through an entire day without worrying about what you can or can't eat.

___ 19. You feel troubled about food or eating, but you don't mention this to others because they wouldn't understand.

___ 20. You're terrified of the scale.

___ 21. You feel fat even though others think you're thin.

___ 22. You don't like your body.

___ 23. You feel that happiness will elude you until you lose weight.

___ 24. You are preoccupied with weight, food, diets, and calories.

___ 25. You get up and eat at night, after everyone has gone to bed.

___ 26. You fast regularly.

___ 27. You make sure to count every calorie.

___ 28. You eat in secret.

___ 29. You regularly perform exhausting exercise routines to burn off the calories you've eaten.

___ 30. You alternate between severely restricting your eating and eating large quantities of food.

___ 31. You've dieted on and off for most of your life.

___ 32. The first thing you think about in the morning is food.

___ 33. You're very afraid of gaining weight and becoming fat.

___ 34. You often eat until you're uncomfortably full.

___ 35. You've had an out-of-control eating binge at least one time in the past year.

___ 36. You panic if you can't exercise to burn off food that you've eaten.

(continued)

__ 37. After a binge, at least one time during the past year you have: made yourself vomit, fasted, used diet pills, exercised excessively, or used laxatives, enemas, diuretics, or colonics.

__ 38. You eat to make yourself feel better emotionally, but it ends up making you feel guilty and depressed.

__ 39. You don't eat much in front of others, but you eat large amounts of food when you're by yourself.

__ 40. You become anxious around food.

To score: For each "true" answer to questions 1 through 23, give yourself 1 point; for each "true" answer to questions 24 through 40, give yourself 2 points.

    0 to 5: You may have a few eating issues, but they probably don't interfere with your life.

    6 to 10: Runaway Eating may be on the horizon.

  11 to 15: You have mild to moderate Runaway Eating.

  16 to 20: Runaway Eating is definitely a problem.

21 and up: In addition to using the self-help strategies in this book, see a physician or mental health professional for help.

CHAPTER 3

What Causes Runaway Eating, and Who's at Risk?

"I've watched my diet and been a faithful exerciser all
my life, and I'm the one who's developed a binge
problem. My best friend, Jan, lives on fried food and
never goes to the gym, yet food has never been an
issue for her. Why did I end up with this problem?"
—Deena, 39-year-old stay-at-home mom

Why me?" That's the question many women who feel out of
control around food ask themselves. After all, you probably
consider yourself successful in other aspects of your life. So why
has food, of all things, become such a big issue for you?

Earlier, we discussed why midlife is such a stressful time for
women and why women tend to turn to food—as an "acceptable"
vice—to comfort or console themselves or just to put off dealing
with their troubles for a few minutes. But if we've all engaged in
emotional eating at some point in our lives, then why do only

some of us become Runaway Eaters? To answer this question, we need to take a closer look at the major factors that put us at risk for Runaway Eating. Although not every one of these may pertain to your unique situation, some will undoubtedly strike a chord.

RISK FACTORS FOR RUNAWAY EATING

The risk factors for Runaway Eating are as wide-ranging as society's insistence on thinness as a prerequisite for female beauty and as personal as a family history of depression. And whether your Runaway Eating takes the form of bingeing, restricting, or bingeing and purging, the driving forces behind these behaviors are basically the same. Just being female predisposes you to eating problems, as does a tendency toward anxiety, perfectionism, self-criticism, and the hormone swings experienced during the years leading up to and following menopause. And though having risk factors for eating problems doesn't ensure that you'll develop Runaway Eating, it does set the stage. It's like gathering a big pile of flammable material. You won't necessarily start a fire, but all it takes is a spark.

The Beauty Factor

Although it is unfair, shallow, and ridiculous, for thousands of years society has measured a woman's worth in terms of her beauty. Those who physically conform most closely to the cultural ideals of their time tend to have easier access to life's goodies: rich, powerful, attractive partners; material goods; career advancement; adulation; acclaim; even love. This is not a new revelation. We're all well aware of the power of beauty, and most of us spend a good deal of our time and money on cosmetics, trips to the hair salon, manicures, and updating our wardrobes to include the latest fashions or this year's color. But one element that society deems necessary for feminine attractiveness carries with it the added wallop of being downright dangerous—that of being thin, skinny, slim, or slender. For most of us, this runs contrary to our genetic legacy, and trying to achieve and maintain an artificially low weight can exact a terrible physical, mental, and emotional price.

To see just how high the "beauty bar" has been raised, let's take a closer look at society's changing standards of beauty in the last century.

The early 1900s: Thin becomes in. In our thinness-obsessed society, it's hard to imagine a time when a fuller figure was the cultural ideal. But during the 18th and 19th centuries, plumpness and soft, feminine curves—including a full bosom and rounded hips—were highly prized characteristics of the sexually attractive woman. They indicated that she came from the well-fed upper class and didn't have to engage in physical labor.

It wasn't until the early 20th century, when food had become much more abundant, that an ample body no longer held sway as a status symbol. Instead, the American upper class began to affect the European ideal of the body beautiful—one that was slim, trim, and slender—to distinguish themselves from the stocky, full-bodied immigrants. Before long, slimness had taken on a whole new meaning. It was a symbol of discipline and good breeding, while heaviness took on the overtones of greediness, laziness, and lack of self-control.

During the early 1900s, Americans fell in love with the Gibson girl, a pen-and-ink drawing of an idealized young woman conjured up by illustrator Charles Dana Gibson. The Gibson girl was the artist's fantasy of the most beautiful girl he could imagine: She was tall, exceedingly slim, and had a fit, athletic body with slightly broad shoulders and a very small waist. She also possessed a gorgeous face. Nobody actually looked like the Gibson girl, because she wasn't real. Yet she captivated the American imagination, and advertisers used her to promote everything from soap to stockings. Then a strange thing happened. Bombarded by images of this fantasy creature, women started to feel bad about their own looks. They measured themselves against this phony standard of beauty and felt inferior. This began a disturbing new trend that exists to this day: Advertisers set the "beauty bar" impossibly high, and women felt self-conscious and inferior because they couldn't reach those unrealistic goals.

Just as the Gibson girl was gaining in popularity, a "physical fitness" craze hit the country, and for the first time, women were trying out sports like cycling and tennis. Calisthenics, including jumping jacks and deep knee bends, were all the rage. Obviously, the long, full skirts and voluminous petticoats that women had been wearing weren't going to work with this new active lifestyle, so skirts were shortened (and sometimes divided), corsets were released, and sleeves were cropped. After hundreds of years of draping their bodies with yards of fabric and relying on foundation garments to augment shape, women found that the outlines of their bodies were suddenly a lot more visible. And they began to feel more self-conscious and more negative about their looks.

The 1920s: The more we reveal, the worse we feel. In the 1920s, the revelation of the body grew even more extreme—as a result of the rebellious flappers who wanted to be free to dance, play sports, and lead much more active lives than women had in the past. Skirts barely scraped the tops of the calves, sleeves disappeared, and corsets were permanently relegated to the attic. In response, women's anxieties about their bodies skyrocketed, setting many on a quest to attain the perfect flapper's body—small, slim, and flat-chested. During the flapper era, dieting became commonplace, with fasting, fad diets, self-induced vomiting, and laxative abuse all popular weight-control methods.

Advertisers were happy to take advantage of women's insecurities about their bodies and widely promoted weight-loss gadgets like reducing belts, creams, weight-loss tonics, stimulating brushes, bath salts, and special diets. Naturally, all of these devices were demonstrated by slim, gorgeous young women. The message was clear: Slim down, and you'll be beautiful and happy.

The 1940s through the 1970s: Thinness becomes a fashion statement. Have you ever wondered why clothing designers always use superthin, even skeletal-looking models to show off their clothes? It began back in the 1940s, when designers discovered that very thin women didn't have the pesky curves that disturbed the way the clothes hung on the body. Thin models were more like hangers, allowing the fabric to fall straight down from their shoulders, skimming the body in clean, unbroken lines. Like a hanger, the model herself became invisible, and the garment took center stage.

At some point, though, the hanger began to take on some of the characteristics of the garments—that is, the superthin body became associated with high-style beauty. In effect, the hanger became an object of beauty in itself. There was only one problem: Hardly anyone had a body that looked like a hanger. Instead of recognizing the ridiculousness of this new gold standard for body types, women tried to force their bodies to conform to these new, thinner ideals. Self-consciousness and self-deprecation increased; diets and other reducing methods followed.

The epitome of the skinny model was a 95-pound, 5-foot-6 teenager named Twiggy, who exploded onto the fashion scene in the late 1960s and was exploited for her emaciation. Measuring

31-22-32, her sticklike figure made everyone feel heavy in comparison, even slim women. To make matters worse, the fashions of the day (including the miniskirt, the bikini, and the topless bathing suit) left very little to the imagination. Diet pills, liquid lunches, and skipped meals all became *de rigueur.*

By the time the 1970s rolled around, America's drive for thinness had reached a fever pitch. The mantra of the day was "You can never be too thin or too rich," a saying that some women even embroidered onto pillows. Eating disorders, conditions that heretofore had been practically unseen, suddenly burst into the public consciousness.

The 1980s: Exercise, exercise, exercise. . . . A huge fitness craze engulfed the nation during the 1980s, with Jane Fonda at the helm, urging women to exercise intensely enough to "feel the burn." Now, not only was a woman supposed to be thin, she was supposed to have well-defined muscles, a flat stomach, and a small, tight derriere. Jane herself provided the ultimate example, with her slim, well-toned, perfectly proportioned figure. (Much later, we learned that Fonda had suffered from bulimia for years.) One small problem: This look was completely out of the realm of possibility for most women. And those who did manage to look like Jane Fonda were only able to do so by spending countless hours at the gym, starving, or purging. The age of excessive exercise was upon us.

The 1990s: Why don't I look like Goldie Hawn? Beginning in the 1990s and continuing into the new century, we've been confronted with yet another impossible standard of beauty: the middle-aged woman who never seems to age. No longer is it just the young who are pressured to conform to unrealistic notions of the body beautiful. The media continually celebrate women who are over 40 but have the body of a 20-year-old—think Goldie

Hawn, Christie Brinkley, Demi Moore, and Michelle Pfeiffer. Thanks to their unusual genetic legacies, round-the-clock personal trainers, and, in some cases, bouts of plastic surgery, these celebrities continue to look like college girls. Yet even though they're anomalies, the widespread publicity they've received has set the beauty bar for midlife women even higher than before— somewhere up there in the stratosphere. The message is clear: Looking normal for your age group is bad, and it's your own fault for not trying harder.

Family Matters

Eating problems tend to run in families, so if one or more of your parents or siblings have issues with food or weight, you're more likely to have them as well. This may be due to genetic factors, environmental stressors, or a dysfunctional family environment. Most likely, all of these influences play a part in the genesis and maintenance of your eating problem. Let's take a look at each.

Genes. Your genetic legacy may play a role in whether you become a Runaway Eater. The families of those with clinically defined eating disorders tend to have high rates of anorexia, bulimia, depression, anxiety, obsessive-compulsive disorders, and other mood disorders. Because a tendency to develop an eating disorder can be passed on genetically, scientists have wondered whether the tendency to develop disturbed eating behavior, such as Runaway Eating, could be passed on genetically as well.

Recent studies on families and twins have shown that the relatives of a person who has an eating disorder are 7 to 12 times more likely to have an eating disorder themselves. But how much of this is due to a shared genetic legacy, and how much has to do with living in an environment that promotes unhealthy eating? It's hard to discern, because the same people who gave you your genes are also the ones responsible for your environment. (Do children with high IQs owe their intellectual excellence to good genes or to parents who have provided them with an enriched environment? And are parents who have intellectually superior genes more likely to provide enriched environments for their kids? It's reminiscent of the old which-came-first—the chicken or the egg?—question.)

As it turns out, research indicates that somewhere between 50 and 80 percent of a person's risk for developing anorexia and bulimia lies in the genes. Still, that leaves environmental factors responsible for a hefty 20 to 50 percent of the risk, a significant portion.

Although researchers are just starting to identify genes that can increase a person's risk of developing anorexia and bulimia, it's a tricky process because eating disorders aren't caused by just one gene gone bad. Instead, they result from a complex interaction between many genetic and environmental factors. For example, let's say that you have certain genes associated with anxiety plus the ability to survive on relatively small amounts of food for a long period of time. During times of famine, these could be valuable adaptive traits that would help you survive. But in modern society, they could increase your risk for developing anorexia nervosa.

Environmental stressors. The wild card in the eating disorder deck is that the genes that put you at risk for developing a problem might become active only when certain environmental stressors are present. You may go for years without ever developing an eating problem; then something happens to set it off. The spark may be something as benign as a wedding or a class reunion. Or it may be something much more serious, such as coping with a divorce or depression, going through menopause, or struggling with chronic work overload.

The one stressor that is seen in practically all cases of problematic eating is unhealthy dieting. Let's say you have the genes mentioned above, which make you tend toward anxiety and able to survive on little food. But you never go on your first radical diet, so these genes never get a chance to express themselves. In contrast, someone else with this same setup, who gets the idea that dieting can help her control her life, begins a strict diet and eventually develops an eating disorder.

Dysfunctional family environment. Whether you develop an eating problem may also have something to do with your family of origin. The seeds are often planted very early in life, emerging later as physical symptoms of emotional turmoil.

If you're a Restricting Runaway Eater, you may have come from a family that placed a premium on control. Other family members may have had perfectionistic or obsessive tendencies. There may have been an unstated rule that certain emotions were forbidden. For example, steam could have been coming out of your ears, but if someone asked you if you were mad, you'd know the proper answer was "No, not me!"

Your parents may have discouraged you from developing a strong sense of independence and wanted to live your life for you. The boundaries between you and your parents may have been blurry, with neither of you clearly understanding where one's responsibilities ended and the other's began. There may have been a great deal of unspoken stress in your parents' marriage, forcing you to serve as a kind of spouse substitute. And chances are that your family was very invested in the way they looked. Good looks, good grooming, fashionable clothes, and generally appearing to be the perfect family may have been major goals in your household.

If you're a Bingeing Runaway Eater, your parents may have been distant and emotionally unavailable, and either or both could have suffered from depression. You may have felt that they expected a lot from you and were critical of your performance and of you personally. Your family may have teased you about your eating, weight, or shape, making you feel self-conscious and insecure.

If you're a Runaway Eater who binges and purges, it's more likely that you came from a chaotic family. Chances are you had at least one family member who had problems with alcohol or other drugs. Family conflict was probably the rule rather than the exception in your childhood home, and at times your family may have been quite disorganized and impulsive. These problems may have been hidden from outsiders, to whom your family appeared to be perfectly happy, or they may have been right out there in the open. Either way, family problems were something you wanted to hide from—and to hide from other people.

Your family may exhibit characteristics from any or all of these categories, or none at all. There is no clear-cut division between the kind of family that produces a Runaway Eater who restricts, for example, and the kind that produces one who purges. And it's certainly possible that your Runaway Eating has nothing whatsoever to do with your family of origin. But in many cases, a dysfunctional family does produce a person who is predisposed to developing an eating problem.

Person to Person: Your Individual Risk Factors

Anybody can fall into Runaway Eating, but if you happen to have certain personal characteristics, you may be more at risk. These include the following:

History of being overweight. If you tend to carry extra weight (even slight amounts), you are probably well acquainted with diets and dieting. The more you've dieted, the slower your metabolism is likely to be, making weight loss even more difficult and frustrating for you. Dieting may also have interfered with your normal hunger and satiety signals, so that you eat in response to cues that have nothing to do with your body's needs. The more difficult it is to lose weight, the more important it may become to you. You may believe that the answer to true happiness lies in getting rid of the extra pounds.

History of anorexia or bulimia nervosa. If you've had an eating disorder in the past, your risk of suffering from an eating problem later in life is increased. Follow-up studies of those who have been treated for anorexia find that complete recovery is uncommon (but possible) and that many women continue to exhibit a preoccupation with food and weight for decades. Studies of women with bulimia done 3 years after treatment found that approximately one-third binged/purged less than once a month, one-third binged/purged on a daily basis, and the remaining third fell somewhere in between.

Low self-esteem. Most Runaway Eaters suffer from low self-esteem and are highly self-critical. They feel badly about themselves and try to get rid of these feelings through unhealthy eating behaviors. A Runaway Eater may diet rigidly because she believes that getting thinner will make her a more valuable and worthwhile person. Or she may focus on one "imperfect" part of her body— say, her thighs—and exercise for hours each day, believing that thin thighs will make her happy. Or she may feel that she's a hopeless case and simply bury her negative feelings in food.

Self-worth tied to good looks and thinness. Runaway Eating is quite common among those whose identities, self-esteem, or careers depend on staying slim and looking good. Models, dancers, and actors are particularly vulnerable, because carrying an extra 5 pounds can mean the difference between getting a job and standing in the unemployment line. Performers also tend to have characteristics that exacerbate eating problems, including perfectionism, competitiveness, self-doubt, depression, and anxiety. But any woman who is very invested in her looks or whose looks fuel her self-esteem is vulnerable to Runaway Eating.

Menopause. The risk of obesity rises in midlife owing to changes in metabolism, hormones, and activity levels. For example, the decline of estrogen causes changes in body composition that increase the overall amount of fatty tissue compared with lean body tissue. Many women also begin to put on weight (and inches) in the abdominal area, as estrogen wanes and testosterone (the male sex hormone) becomes more prominent, making the pattern of fat deposition more like a man's. So you might discover unwelcome increases in both your weight and waistline, even when your eating habits stay the same. Further, decreases in estrogen levels are related to increases in appetite, blood sugar fluctuations, and a decreased ability to taste sweetness—all of which can add up to a stronger desire to eat (especially sweets). Fluctuations in hormones can also contribute to anxiety, depression, irritability, hot flashes, insomnia, and a host of other symptoms that make many women more likely to turn to food for comfort, relief, or distraction.

Depression. Research shows that those with eating problems tend to be depressed and that appetite changes and weight fluctuations caused by depression are often key factors in activating and maintaining Runaway Eating. One in five women can expect to develop clinical depression during her lifetime, a condition that often comes in conjunction with anxiety, irritability, fatigue, a sense of hopelessness, and major changes in eating habits. Signs of depression include sadness, persistently low mood for at least 2 weeks, lack of pleasure or interest in usual activities, sleep disturbances, early-morning awakening, appetite disturbances, loss of interest in sex, trouble concentrating, memory problems, and thoughts of suicide.

Anxiety. Some 80 to 90 percent of food binges are triggered by anxiety and tension. We can see this in the Restricting Runaway Eater, who may try to relieve stress by not eating and whose stress levels skyrocket when she breaks a dietary rule. For this type of person, controlling food intake, even to the point of starvation, may actually reduce her baseline anxiety level. On the other hand, the Bingeing Runaway Eater uses eating sprees as a way to seek relief from anxiety. She temporarily lets go of strict dietary regimens or uses food as an instantaneous way to calm or distract herself. Then there's the Bingeing/Compensating Runaway Eater, who falls off her diet and experiences intense anxiety until she gets rid of those extra calories, either by purging or overexercising. Many Runaway Eaters live in a perpetual state of anxiety, afraid of food, of gaining weight, of not being good enough, and even of their own bodies.

Perfectionism. Most Runaway Eaters are perfectionists, demanding 110 percent from themselves. But no matter how much they achieve, they never seem to be satisfied. They are highly competitive, become extremely distressed about any mistakes they make, and are subject to high levels of self-doubt. Perfectionism may work together with body dissatisfaction and low self-esteem to bring on Runaway Eating. Although there exists a healthy drive for success, in which an individual sets realistic goals and is motivated by the rewards and pleasures associated with succeeding, the Runaway Eater is usually involved in a more extreme type of perfectionism that is unhealthy. She sets extremely high, unrealistic goals for herself and is driven by a fear of failure. To her, mistakes are synonymous with disaster.

Poor problem-solving skills. Runaway Eaters tend to have

difficulty solving their problems because they aren't able to address their difficulties head on. Thus, the woman who is depressed because her marriage is troubled may "solve" the problem by going on a diet and losing 20 pounds. Or the stressed-out working mother whose boss is angry because she can't work overtime may eat an entire box of cookies at night to relieve the tension. A Runaway Eater typically tries to avoid confrontation and may feel as if her own point of view isn't worthy of being heard. So eating or eating-related behaviors become her response to emotional upsets, instead of dealing with those emotional upsets directly.

Other personality factors. Generally, the Restricting Runaway Eater tends to be aloof, withdrawn, and somewhat lonely, almost as if she were starving herself of affection. She is highly perfectionistic, disciplined, and self-controlled. She also tends to be socially self-conscious and very sensitive to the opinions of others. Her mistrust of others leads her to try hard to control them. She often feels undeserving of food or positive things in life.

The Bingeing/Compensating Runaway Eater, on the other hand, alternates between being overcontrolled and undercontrolled. Her life resembles a roller coaster. She is also much more likely to abuse drugs or other substances, or get involved in unhealthy relationships. She always seems to be on a diet, but she can't make herself stay with it for long. Her bingeing and purging are sometimes exhibited in her personal relationships as well as in her food behaviors. For example, she may have very intense relationships in which she gets overly attached to a person. But soon she gets fed up with the person and has an overwhelming urge to "get rid" of him or her.

The Bingeing Runaway Eater shares some of the personality features of the Bingeing/Compensating Runaway Eater, although she doesn't try to compensate for her binges. She tends to be highly concerned about her weight and appearance and feels shameful, inadequate, and worthless because her body seems to be all wrong. She tends to be anxious and may avoid social occasions, especially the kind involving food. Her all-or-nothing thinking can bring on binges whenever she goes off her diet even slightly or feels anxious, depressed, or in need of comfort. But she also tends to overeat outside of her binges, often consuming unusually large meals and snacking excessively. Bingeing Runaway Eaters can be worriers, and worrying can fuel their binges. They are often fatigued and can be plagued with multiple aches and pains.

THE CATALYST: DIETING

All of us live in a society where looksism is rampant. Many people come from troubled families, and a lot of them experience anxiety, depression, or low self-esteem at one time or another. Some of us even have a genetic predisposition to an eating problem. Yet not all of us become Runaway Eaters. What makes one person turn to a destructive eating behavior while another with a similar setup doesn't fall into the trap?

The answer, in many cases, is dieting. Most Runaway Eating begins with an old friend, the seemingly innocent diet. You may think that dieting is good for you—that it's the one thing that stands between you and obesity. It may even seem to be a morally and ethically responsible choice—after all, aren't we supposed to take charge of our bodies and our health? And these days, following the latest diet trend can even be fashionable; witness the immense recent popularity of the low-carb diets! But the truth is that intentional attempts to restrict your food intake are bad for both your body and your mind. Besides the fact that diets are ineffective—95 percent of those who go on a diet eventually gain the weight back, plus a few pounds—they also promote Runaway Eating by:

- Encouraging rigid, hypercontrolled behavior
- Promoting poor self-esteem, depression, and isolation
- Slowing metabolism, making it even more difficult to maintain a healthy body weight
- Encouraging obsessive thoughts and behaviors regarding eating
- Promoting an all-or-nothing attitude
- Interfering with the body's natural hunger and satiety (fullness) signals
- Triggering binges
- Ensuring that you, the dieter, will eventually fail, which can trigger even more restrictive and dangerous weight-loss strategies

Any and all of these attitudes or behaviors will feed directly into the Runaway Eating cycle. And once the cycle begins, dieting only serves to reinforce the Runaway Eating behaviors.

Are All Diets Unhealthy?

Want the short answer? *Yes.* Now, you may be thinking, "If I don't stay on some kind of diet, I'll just blow up like a balloon. I need to be on a program just to keep control of myself." But consider that any kind of dieting involves a diet mentality, which ensures failure, encourages you to ignore hunger and satiety signals, and promotes a negative relationship with food, because you have to give up "forbidden" foods and, often, eat foods you don't really like. This inevitably results in giving in, which often means binge-ing and feeling terrible about yourself. So, though this idea may sound radical, we firmly believe there is *no* good diet.

By "diet," we mean the conscious restriction of the amounts or kind of foods you're allowed to eat for the express purpose of losing weight. A diet is something that you go on when you want to change your body, and go off once you've reached a certain goal. Though we certainly do endorse consuming a wide variety of healthful foods, paying attention to portion sizes, and thinking twice before eating a lot of foods that are high in calories but low in nutrition, we don't recommend following any kind of plan that tells you what, how much, and how often you should eat, without regard for your body's hunger and satiety signals. And we definitely don't recommend any eating plan that you go on and then go off.

Although it may sound surprising, the negative effects of dieting also hold true even if you aren't following a formal diet but still think like a dieter. If you count grams of fat, opt for high-protein foods while shunning carbs, rely on "safe" foods, beat yourself up for eating "bad" foods, consciously or unconsciously undereat (which can trigger overeating later), use diet soft drinks or coffee to quell your hunger, or decide what you can eat based on what you've already eaten today, you're dieting.

In chapter 5, we'll discuss how you can teach yourself to once again recognize and listen to your body's hunger and satiety signals. We'll also teach you how to make peace with food, which means eating foods that honor both your health and your taste-buds. For now, though, simply understanding the harmful effects of dieting is a crucial step.

The Physical and Psychological Effects of Dieting

Have you ever noticed that as soon as you go on a diet, all you want to do is eat? Even if you weren't particularly concerned about food prior to dieting, all of a sudden you become obsessed with it. You find yourself preoccupied with what you'll have for your next meal, whether you can have a snack, what others are eating, or even what you'll allow yourself to eat tomorrow. What's going on?

The mind and the body are inextricably linked, and never is this more apparent than when you go on a diet. Geared to survive during feast or famine, both body and mind switch into survival mode when the food supply is radically diminished. While the body turns down the metabolism and becomes a "slow burner" in an attempt to hang on to every single calorie, the mind gears itself to one overriding purpose: getting food. The result? Suddenly, you may find yourself clipping recipes, planning menus, cooking elaborate meals or dishes for others (neither of which you'll eat yourself), or even dreaming about food at night. The message is clear: Your body wants food, and your mind does, too.

After a few days of extremely restricting your food, you'll probably become more depressed and anxious. Although this may be due to changes in neurotransmitters like serotonin, it may also occur because you are depriving yourself of things that are very pleasurable that aren't replaced by anything else—leaving a pleasure void. You may suddenly prefer to spend more time alone—it takes too much energy to deal with others—and your self-esteem may start to drop. Unfortunately, the more depressed, anxious, and isolated you become, the more you'll obsess about food.

Some people can hold out longer than others, but the result is eventually the same: a binge. You eat something you "shouldn't," which makes you feel as if you've blown it. So you let go and eat. During the binge you feel relief—at last you can relax and do what you've wanted to do all along. But you may also feel as if you're in a trance and can't stop yourself. It's almost as if your body has developed a will of its own; it's going to feed itself whether you like it or not. As a result, you can end up eating more food in one sitting than you ever did when you weren't dieting.

Are you crazy? Absolutely not. This is a normal, even healthy reaction to a period of semi-starvation, a reaction that made good sense during primitive times. After a period of famine, it was natural and necessary for our ancient ancestors to overeat. They needed to be able to take advantage of a feast when they had the chance, because the food supply was uncertain. To make this possible, their appetites increased after a period of famine. So the same amount of food that would have satisfied them during times of plenty left them feeling hungry after a period of semi-starvation. The same thing happens to you when you restrict food. Suddenly, you develop the urge and the capacity to binge, and you no longer feel satisfied after eating what you used to consider a normal meal. In short, *restrictive dieting can trigger binges and leave you hungry even after you've eaten normal amounts of food.* This is true for most Runaway Eaters, and even for those dieters who do not develop Runaway Eating problems.

The psychological consequences of dieting were clearly illustrated in a classic study of the effects of semi-starvation done in 1950 by Ancel Keys, Ph.D., and his colleagues at the University of Minnesota. In the study, 36 healthy, young, psychologically sound males were observed over a period of 1 year. During the first 3 months, the men ate normal amounts of food; during the next 6 months, they were given half as much food; and during the last 3 months, their food allotment was gradually increased. During the semi-starvation period, the men became preoccupied with food and constantly talked about it, read cookbooks, clipped recipes, and daydreamed about eating. When a meal was served, many took an inordinately long time to eat it, trying to make it last. Over time, the men became extremely depressed, anxious, and irritable.

Once they made it through the period of semi-starvation, the men ate nearly continuously, with some indulging in 8,000- to 10,000-calorie binges. The men reported that their hunger actually *increased* right after meals, and some of them continued to eat to the point of being sick without feeling satisfied. Although most of the men finally reverted to normal eating patterns within 5 months of the study's end, some continued with their new patterns of "extreme overconsumption."

We see these same patterns in dieters: the preoccupation with food; the anxiety, depression, and irritability; the tendency to go off the diet and eat more than one would have in the pre-diet days; and a propensity toward bingeing even after the diet has ended.

Hunger and Satiety: The On/Off Eating Switches

As we've seen, two of the body's most important survival mechanisms are hunger (which tells you it's time to eat) and satiety (a feeling of fullness and satisfaction that tells you it's time to stop eating). When you were a baby, you knew when and how much you needed to eat, and you let your mother know in no uncertain terms. But dieting trains you to ignore both hunger and satiety, causing you to eventually lose touch with these important signals. Diets, by definition, dictate what, how much, and when you should eat, and your success as a dieter is primarily dependent upon your being able to ignore your natural instincts. You learn to restrain your appetite when you're hungry, and when you have a rebound binge, you simply power right through those fullness signals. But by overriding your natural instincts time after time, you eventually unlearn what you knew as an infant, and you can end up eating much more or much less than you should. Thus, the Restricting

DO LOW-CARB DIETS ENCOURAGE BINGEING?

According to Christopher Fairburn, M.D., of Oxford University, the nutritional composition of food has an important influence on appetite control. One effect of eating carbohydrates, he says, is their rapid and potent suppression of hunger. He warns that people who avoid foods that contain carbohydrates are denying themselves a natural appetite suppressant.

What's the link between appetite suppression and carbs? Normally, after you've consumed a certain amount of food, the neurotransmitter serotonin trips a "satiety switch" in your brain, letting you know it's time to stop eating. But the amount of serotonin that's produced in your brain is affected by the amount of carbohydrates you consume. So if you follow a diet that has you restricting carbs, your serotonin levels could diminish. The result? You may never receive the "stop eating" message.

Bingeing can also be triggered by an increased appetite for carbohydrates, a common occurrence when carbs are restricted. Studies with rats given a high-protein, low-carbohydrate diet for 3 weeks showed that when starch was reintroduced into their diets, they ate not only significantly more carbohydrates than a control group but also significantly more total food.

Even though one of the so-called pluses of the low-carb diet is that you can eat as much as you want of "approved" foods like meat, cheese, or other high-protein and high-fat foods, these won't satisfy you if you're really craving carbohydrates. According to MIT researcher Judith Wurtman, eating protein or fat when your body is asking for carbs won't quell your craving—it will simply make you tired, apathetic, and lethargic.

Runaway Eater may feel bloated and uncomfortable after eating one piece of bread, while the Bingeing/Compensating Runaway Eater won't feel satisfied even after eating an entire chocolate cake.

How does this happen? In the case of the Restricting Runaway

Eater, existing in a chronic state of semi-starvation will cause her stomach to empty at a much slower rate so that whatever food she does eat can be absorbed more efficiently. As a result, one piece of bread can take longer to digest, causing an uncomfortable feeling of fullness. In the case of the Runaway Eater who binges and purges, dieting may alter the level of certain critical brain chemicals (such as serotonin) that would normally signal fullness. Diets that restrict certain food groups (like carbohydrates) may also influence the levels of these brain chemicals. Because she doesn't get that "Ah, I've had enough" satisfied feeling of fullness, the Runaway Eater may continue to eat until her stomach simply can't hold any more.

A NO-WIN SITUATION:
THE RUNAWAY EATING MERRY-GO-ROUND

As we've seen, Runaway Eating is the result of a complex combination of factors that trigger unhealthy eating behaviors. One way to visualize Runaway Eating is as a never-ending cycle of thoughts, feelings, and behaviors that feed into each other and result in unhealthy eating behaviors. We've dubbed this process the Runaway Eating merry-go-round, and it's a vicious circle that gets stronger, more destructive, and more entrenched over time. It has five distinct parts.

- ◆ Situational triggers, which promote . . .
- ◆ Destructive thinking, which increases . . .
- ◆ Stress, which triggers . . .
- ◆ Unhealthy eating-related behaviors, which bring on . . .
- ◆ Negative emotions

THE RUNAWAY EATING MERRY-GO-ROUND

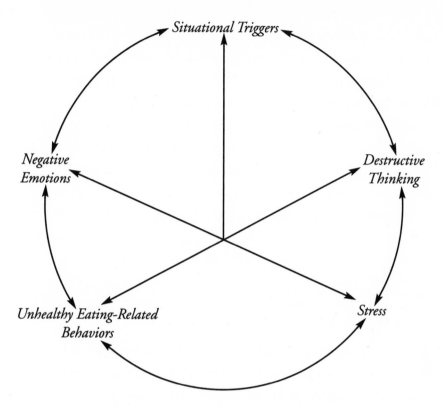

Situational Triggers

Negative Emotions

Destructive Thinking

Unhealthy Eating-Related Behaviors

Stress

The negative emotions then restart the cycle by making the situational triggers even more powerful, which prompt even more destructive thinking.

How does it work? Let's take, for example, a person who has decided that her weight and her eating habits have rendered her life out of control. We'll call her Susan. She believes that if she can just take charge of her food and weight issues, she will regain control of her life. Susan is also at risk of developing eating problems for various other reasons that may be rooted in her background.

Let's say that her mother had an eating problem, and she herself has a history of being overweight, leans toward depression, suffers from bouts of anxiety, and has perfectionistic tendencies. Susan's excess weight bothers her greatly; she wants to look "right," and to her that means losing at least 20 pounds. She is a prime candidate for Runaway Eating, but first something has to set her off.

Situational triggers. The "something" that sets off Susan's Runaway Eating may be an upcoming class reunion, a wedding, seeing a picture of herself that she thinks makes her look fat, a tactless comment someone makes about her appearance, or her own impending divorce. Society's oppressive emphasis on thinness certainly contributes. But whatever the trigger may be, something in her environment trips the switch that increases her feelings of anxiety, inferiority, depression, or self-consciousness about not being good enough. She decides to go on a diet, take back control of her life, and lose the weight for good.

Destructive thinking. Susan begins a strict diet and sternly tells herself that this time there will be no fooling around. She insists that she must follow the diet perfectly and doesn't allow herself to take even one bite of any "forbidden foods." She may also force herself to perform a long, exhausting exercise routine. But then comes the inevitable moment when she slips up and overeats, or misses an exercise session, which unleashes a torrent of self-criticism, and her weakened self-esteem plunges.

Stress. Susan's stress levels skyrocket, thanks to her self-punishing behaviors, negative self-talk, and difficult diet and exercise regimens. She becomes depressed, anxious, and exhausted and may suffer from insomnia or headaches. She stays away from other people, which depresses her even further, and her thinking becomes distorted. Her body becomes the enemy in the war she's waging.

Unhealthy eating-related behaviors. With her stress levels ratcheted up to the breaking point, Susan feels she has to do some-thing, and her response will dictate the form that her Runaway Eating takes. She may restrict her food intake even more or in-crease her exercise to unhealthy levels. Or, more likely, she may fall into bingeing, or bingeing and purging. Or she may combine these behaviors. But no matter which route she takes, the result will be the same: She'll be hit with a torrent of negative emotions.

Negative emotions. Whether Susan restricts, exercises exces-sively, abuses laxatives or diuretics, binges, or binges and purges, she is awash in depression, guilt, anxiety, self-hatred, fear, and low self-esteem. The out-of-control feelings that began the cycle have now become even worse, and she feels more stressed and frantic to control herself than she did when she started. To make matters worse, her sensitivity to environmental triggers has now increased. Going to the movies and looking at the slim, beautiful actresses on the screen or pulling on a pair of too-tight jeans can be all it takes to set her off on yet another round.

As time goes on, any of the elements of the Runaway Eating merry-go-round can trigger any of the others. For example, de-structive thinking can intensify negative emotions, and situational triggers can heighten stress. Once the Runaway Eating merry-go-round is in motion, it's very difficult to stop. But it can be done—and the rest of this book will show you how.

GETTING OFF THE MERRY-GO-ROUND

If you've found yourself trapped on the Runaway Eating merry-go-round, the first and most important thing you must do is to stop dieting. Fad diets are ineffective and dangerous. Unhealthy dieting not only causes Runaway Eating, destructive emotions, poor concentration, distorted thinking, and a lowered metabolism, but it also assaults your body, mind, and emotions in countless other ways. It sets you up for failure, which can encourage even-more-desperate weight-loss measures.

But what about all the other elements that keep Runaway Eating in business—the depression, the anxiety, the distorted thinking, the perfectionism? All of these will be addressed in detail in the chapters to follow. By following our 8-point plan for conquering Runaway Eating, you'll learn how to overcome problem eating; deal with anxiety, depression, and perfectionism; think about food and eating in new, healthier ways; and eat normally. You'll say goodbye to diets forever and learn to rely on your body's own natural hunger and satiety signals. Your days as a Runaway Eater are about to end.

Part Two

THE 8-POINT PLAN TO CONQUER RUNAWAY EATING

CHAPTER 4

Getting Started:
An Overview

"You have to figure out whether you want your life to be taken over by an obsession. And food *is* an obsession, whether you're stuffing it or restricting it."
—Eliza, 39-year-old preschool teacher

In part one, we discussed the types of Runaway Eating, who's at risk, and the complex array of factors responsible for its growing incidence in recent years. We've seen how Runaway Eating can leave us feeling powerless, frustrated, and exhausted. Somehow, the simple act of feeding ourselves has become a source of anxiety and conflict.

Yet there is hope. It *is* possible to enjoy our meals once again, to eat without feeling guilty, to address the underlying causes behind our Runaway Eating, and to find healthier, more effective ways to deal with them. In the following chapters, you'll discover simple, effective strategies you can use to overcome Runaway Eating—and to regain control of your life.

THE 8-POINT PLAN TO REIN IN
RUNAWAY EATING

Our 8-point plan is designed to conquer Runaway Eating by attacking it at its roots, exploring and correcting the conditions that promote problematic eating behaviors and that keep them functioning. The 8 steps are:

Step 1: Eat on time and in time.
Step 2: Identify your triggers.
Step 3: Reroute your thinking.
Step 4: Transform your moods.
Step 5: Alleviate anxiety.
Step 6: Defuse depression.
Step 7: Manage your menopausal symptoms.
Step 8: Pare down perfectionism.

We certainly don't guarantee that by following this program you'll end up looking like Goldie Hawn—and that shouldn't be your goal. But we do believe that it can change your life. By addressing the driving forces behind problematic eating, our 8-point program can help you regain control over your eating, your body, and your life. Keep in mind that there are no short-term fixes for Runaway Eating; this plan is designed for the long term. Also, be aware that not all of these steps may be relevant for you, though most will be, and you're free to pick and choose the ones that strike a chord.

Before you begin, it's important that you have a thorough consultation with your physician, as it's possible that your eating problems may be rooted in some kind of physical trouble, including a hormonal problem, metabolic condition, cancer, severe depression that can influence your appetite, or a neurological problem such as a seizure disorder. Take this book with you and tell your doctor that you're thinking about beginning the program we describe; explain that you'd like a general examination and any relevant lab work before doing so. Remember that any physical problems must be resolved before you begin this program.

A CLOSER LOOK AT THE 8 STEPS

Based on the success these strategies have had in clinical practice, we believe that the Runaway Eating plan is the single most effective approach to dealing with problematic eating behaviors, particularly those that affect so many women in midlife. Below is a short explanation of each step; detailed discussions will follow in the chapters to come.

Step I: Eat on Time and in Time

Believe it or not, the best way to avoid problematic eating is to eat, regularly and nonemotionally. Don't wait until you're starving and out of control. Eating regularly and learning to reestablish and trust your body's hunger and satiety signals are important first steps toward banishing Runaway Eating.

In chapter 5, we'll show you how to embrace Enjoyable Eating. You'll make peace with food, eat what you really like in sensible quantities (while enjoying it to the hilt), avoid eating in response to emotions, and make food choices that are good for both your health and your tastebuds. Enjoyable Eating will do much to lower the anxiety and depression that accompany dieting, to eliminate bingeing, to increase your self-confidence, and to improve your relationship with food. Ultimately, this can and does result in weight loss, although that should not be your primary goal.

MEDICATIONS FOR EATING PROBLEMS

If you follow our 8-point plan for several months and find that you're still wrestling with eating problems, you might want to ask your doctor about taking medication, which can help correct a biological system that has lost its center. In severe cases of Runaway Eating, your doctor may prescribe medications to help manage coexisting conditions, like depression or anxiety, or to regulate your hunger and satiety signals. None of these medications has been shown to cure eating disorders, but they may help manage symptoms.

Prozac

Generic name: Fluoxetine hydrochloride

Prescribed for: Depression, obsessive-compulsive disorder, bulimia nervosa

How it works: Prozac, which belongs to a class of antidepressants called the selective serotonin reuptake inhibitors (SSRIs), is currently the only medication approved by the FDA for the treatment of eating disorders (specifically bulimia nervosa). Prozac and other SSRIs work by increasing the amount of sero-

tonin available in the brain. This helps to slow the binge-and-purge cycle, while treating coexisting depression, obsessive-compulsive disorder, and panic disorder.

Other SSRIs commonly prescribed for eating problems include the following:

Luvox

Generic name: Fluvoxamine maleate

Prescribed for: Depression and obsessive-compulsive disorder

How it works: Luvox interferes with the uptake of serotonin in the brain, making this neurotransmitter more available to interact with target nerves. It can be used to treat obsessive-compulsive disorder, major depression, and panic disorder and may assist with decreasing the frequency of bingeing and purging.

Paxil

Generic name: Paroxetine hydrochloride

Prescribed for: Serious depression

How it works: Paxil helps slow the binge-and-purge cycle, while treating coexisting depression, obsessive-compulsive disorder, and panic disorder by increasing the amount of serotonin in the brain.

Zoloft

Generic name: Sertraline hydrochloride

Prescribed for: Major depression, obsessive-compulsive disorder, panic disorder (with or without agoraphobia)

How it works: Zoloft prevents serotonin uptake in the brain, increasing its available amounts. It is used to treat depression, obsessive-compulsive disorder, and panic disorder and can help slow the binge-and-purge cycle.

Other medications used to treat eating problems include the following:

Topamax

Generic name: Topiramate

Prescribed for: The treatment of epilepsy (FDA approved). Although topiramate is an anticonvulsant, it is also being studied as a treatment for obsessive-compulsive disorder and is used to treat binge-eating, though it is not officially approved for these purposes.

How it works: Topiramate interferes with the glutamate system in the brain. When glutamate, an amino acid, is injected into animals, their appetites increase markedly and they eat ferociously. By acting as an antagonist to the glutamate system, topiramate may regulate appetite, causing weight loss and decreasing the desire to binge.

Zofran

Generic name: Ondansetron

Prescribed for: Prevention of nausea and vomiting caused by radiation therapy and chemotherapy for cancer. Zofran has also shown promise as a treatment for bulimia.

How it works: Zofran calms the vagus nerve, which extends from the brain stem through organs in the neck, thorax, and abdomen. This nerve controls feelings of satiety after eating. Researchers believe that the constant stimulation of bingeing and purging may damage the vagus nerve, making it unable to trigger a feeling of fullness that leads to meal termination. By calming the vagus nerve, Zofran may help to reinstate normal feelings of satisfaction and fullness after meals.

Step 2: Identify Your Triggers

To get off the Runaway Eating merry-go-round, you must first learn to identify the internal and external cues that lead to unhealthy eating. What is making you eat (or restrict or purge or exercise excessively)? What functions do your unhealthy eating behaviors serve in your life? (One of the big "advantages" of focusing on food, weight, and food-related behaviors is that you don't have time to focus on the underlying troubles in your life.)

In chapter 6, you'll explore how and why your Runaway Eating evolved and how eating behaviors serve a specific nonfood function in your life. You will also learn how certain thoughts, especially untrue beliefs we call Thought Myths, can trigger feelings and behaviors that set off the Runaway Eating cycle and keep it going.

Step 3: Reroute Your Thinking

Runaway Eating takes root when you think about food and weight in distorted ways. You may find yourself attributing special, unwarranted powers to food, food-related behaviors, or weight. For example, you may think, "If I can just lose 15 pounds, my husband will love me more." Or "If I eat this candy bar, I'll feel happy." Or "If I can follow my diet perfectly for one whole week, I'll know that I'm in control of my life." These Thought Myths do much to keep destructive eating habits in play. To stop Runaway Eating, you must learn to banish your Thought Myths and think about food and weight in completely new ways.

In chapter 7, we'll help you to identify the Thought Myths you may have unwittingly adopted, and discuss how to replace them with healthier, more realistic thoughts.

Step 4: Transform Your Moods

Runaway Eaters tend to rely heavily on food or food-related behaviors to regulate their moods, but this isn't an effective strategy. That's because most bad moods, such as sadness, anger, frustration, and irritation, are the result of low levels of energy and high levels of tension. When your energy flags and tension gets the upper hand, you may experience physical and emotional symptoms including knotted muscles, tooth grinding, headaches, fatigue, or a down feeling, all of which can prompt Runaway Eating behaviors. But it's not the food you're after—what you're really looking for is a boost in energy and a release of tension.

In chapter 8, we'll present the results of a study on mood-regulating behaviors, which can help you discover the kinds of behaviors that can vault you out of a bad mood most effectively. We also explain which behaviors are best at raising energy and lowering tension levels. Using these lists, you can construct your own list of Mood Transformers—mood-regulating behaviors that are effective substitutes for Runaway Eating.

Step 5: Alleviate Anxiety

We're nervous, fearful, tense, restless, and uneasy, and it's no wonder! We raise children, care for ailing parents, work full-time, handle finances, run a household (perhaps without the help of a mate), deal with menopause, and feel pressure to look young, sexy, and beautiful—all at the same time. Experts estimate that 80 to 90 percent of food binges are brought on by anxiety and tension, and clinical studies show that over half of the people who have anorexia, and many of those with bulimia, have had some kind of anxiety disorder at some point during their lifetime.

Chapter 9 focuses on anxiety and the many techniques you can use to relieve it, including aerobic exercise, relaxation techniques, strategies for simplifying your life, ways to ensure a good night's sleep, and the use of various supplements.

Step 6: Defuse Depression

Research shows that those who have eating problems tend to be depressed and that appetite changes or weight fluctuations caused by depression are often key factors in activating and maintaining unhealthy eating behaviors.

If you're depressed or suffering from problematic eating, chances are that the neurochemical systems in your brain aren't functioning well—especially those related to serotonin, a neurotransmitter that plays an important part in appetite regulation and mood. Fortunately, you don't need to fall into destructive eating behaviors to raise your serotonin levels and ease depression. In chapter 10, we'll present many natural ways to fight depression, including moderate exercise, dietary choices, bright-light therapy, and cognitive-behavioral therapy, as well as the use of certain popular supplements.

Step 7: Manage Your Menopausal Symptoms

Beginning 2 to 8 years before your final period and continuing at least a year afterward (a time span known as perimenopause), the delicate balance between your female hormones becomes upset, which can bring on bouts of anxiety, depression, and irritability. To complicate matters further, your metabolism may slow during this time, the pounds may pile on, your shape may change, you may retain water, you may have trouble with blood sugar swings, and hot flashes and night sweats may interrupt your sleep. Feeling bloated, tired, sad, and anxious, you're much more likely to fall into unhealthy behaviors like Runaway Eating, especially if you're already inclined in that direction.

In chapter 11, we'll detail the many ways of managing menopausal symptoms naturally, which include dietary changes, exercise, and the use of supplements or natural progesterone.

Step 8: Pare Down Perfectionism

Perfectionism is not about doing a good job—it's about trying to do an impossible job. A person with Runaway Eating is often a perfectionist in many areas of her life, but particularly with regard to socially prescribed standards of how she should look. Her self-esteem is tied to her weight or body shape, and she sets unreasonably high dieting and weight-loss goals. She puts great pressure on herself to achieve these goals, but one little slip in her diet or one missed exercise session and she feels like a complete failure. To overcome Runaway Eating, you must first overcome the perfectionism that drives the disorder. And that takes practice. Chapter 12 includes exercises and suggestions that can help you scale back your tendency toward perfectionism.

———— ⚭ ————

There are no magic cures for Runaway Eating, but following our 8-point plan will help you take back control of your life. Developing new, healthier attitudes toward your body and food will be possible, however, only if you treat it as a long-term project. Given time, though, you can beat Runaway Eating and live a life free of obsessions with food, diet, and weight. Congratulations! You've already taken the first step.

CHAPTER 5

Eat on Time and in Time

B elieve it or not, the best way to recover from Runaway Eating is to eat! Or, more accurately, to eat balanced, wholesome meals and snacks spread throughout the day. The opposite approach—dieting, skipping meals, fasting, or otherwise trying to manipulate your food intake—hinders your body's hunger and satiety (fullness) signals, slows your metabolism (which can lead to weight gain), encourages bingeing, and impairs intellectual and emotional function. (Have you ever noticed how difficult it is to make rational decisions when you're hungry?)

To recover from Runaway Eating, you must first heal your body and your mind by consuming a sufficient number of calories in the form of consistent, healthful meals every single day. If you ignore this rule, it can be practically impossible to rid yourself of eating problems.

Eating regular meals and snacks helps to:

- Decrease or eliminate the urge to binge
- Normalize hunger and satiety signals
- Accelerate your metabolic rate (the speed at which you burn calories)
- Stabilize your weight

- Regulate water balance (which eases water retention)
- Ease depression, anxiety, and irritability related to lack of food
- Improve concentration
- Increase energy

But what is healthy eating anyway? After prolonged periods of bingeing, purging, fasting, or following fad diets, many of us no longer know. To make matters more confusing, *healthy eating* is a nebulous term: What's healthy for a 4-foot-10 female data processor is certainly not healthy for a 6-foot-5 male football player. So how do you know what and how much you should be eating every day?

To answer that question, we'll define healthy eating in the sections to follow in terms of what to eat, when to eat, and how to eat—all key factors in controlling Runaway Eating.

WHAT TO EAT

The U.S. Government's Food Guide Pyramid will help you figure out what you need to eat to maintain good health, no matter what your size, shape, or sex. Though the creators of some fad diets have questioned the Food Guide Pyramid's recommendations, the truth is that the pyramid remains a solid and reliable guide to healthy eating. It may look like a diet, but the Food Guide Pyramid is actually just the opposite. A diet tells you the maximum amount of food you should have, whereas the Food Guide Pyramid tells you what you should be eating each day *as a minimum*. It also helps you plan healthful meals by categorizing foods according to group and defining an average serving size of each.

Following is a description of each group, plus the recom-

FOOD GUIDE PYRAMID
A Guide to Daily Food Choices

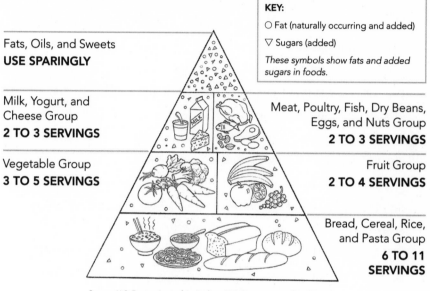

KEY:

○ Fat (naturally occurring and added)

▽ Sugars (added)

These symbols show fats and added sugars in foods.

Fats, Oils, and Sweets
USE SPARINGLY

Milk, Yogurt, and Cheese Group
2 TO 3 SERVINGS

Meat, Poultry, Fish, Dry Beans, Eggs, and Nuts Group
2 TO 3 SERVINGS

Vegetable Group
3 TO 5 SERVINGS

Fruit Group
2 TO 4 SERVINGS

Bread, Cereal, Rice, and Pasta Group
6 TO 11 SERVINGS

Source: U.S. Department of Agriculture/U.S. Department of Health and Human Services, August 1992

mended range of daily servings. You can (and should) eat foods in each group that you really like, and you should vary your food choices within the groups. The basic idea is to eat the bulk of your foods from the grain group (bread, cereal, rice, and pasta). Then add plenty of vegetables and fruits, plus 2 to 3 servings from both the dairy and the protein groups. Finally, add in small amounts of fats, oils, and sweets.

Grains (bread, cereal, rice, and pasta). Get 6 to 11 servings per day.

Serving size: One grain serving is the equivalent of ½ cup of cooked cereal, pasta, or rice or one slice of bread.

Tip: A serving of rice, pasta, or cooked cereal is about the size of your fist. To count as just 1 serving, a roll or muffin should be about the size of a doorknob (those gigantic muffins sold in a lot of bakeries and restaurants are easily 2 or more servings!), and a slice of bread, about the size of a CD.

Grains provide complex carbohydrates, which your body breaks down into glucose, or blood sugar, and uses as fuel. They also provide B vitamins and fiber. As you no doubt know, carbohydrates are currently out of favor in the diet world and are believed to be a big reason that Americans are getting fatter and fatter. This may be true of the refined carbohydrates, like those contained in white flour, sugar, cakes, cookies, candy, and soft drinks. But complex carbohydrates, like those in vegetables, fruits, and whole grains, are actually quite low in calories. (The most fattening part is usually the high-fat spreads or sauces we top them with.) Plus, they help stabilize blood sugar levels and increase production of serotonin, a neurotransmitter that plays an important part in satisfying the appetite.

Whenever possible, choose the complex carbohydrates in whole grains over the simple carbs in refined grains and sugary treats. Refined carbohydrates lead to rapid peaks in blood glucose. When glucose levels fall soon afterward, it can trigger bingeing, depression, and irritability. Whole grains like brown rice, whole wheat, and oats are your best bet for nutrients, fiber, and stabilization of blood glucose.

Fruits and vegetables. Get 2 to 4 servings of fruits and 3 to 5 servings of vegetables per day.

Serving size: One serving equals 1 cup of chopped, raw vegetables or fruit; one medium-size fruit; or ½ cup of fruit or vegetable juice.

Tip: One cup of chopped fruit or vegetables is about the size of a baseball.

Vegetables and fruits provide beta-carotene, vitamin C, fiber, folate, and various disease-fighting substances called phytochemicals. Eat your fruits and vegetables raw, if possible. Limit fruit juice or vegetable juice to 1 serving a day and eat a protein-containing food (like a piece of cheese) along with it to help slow the increase in blood glucose. Also, make sure that your fruit juice is 100 percent fruit juice and doesn't contain sugar or grape juice concentrate, apple juice concentrate, or high-fructose corn syrup, which are all extremely high in sugar.

Protein (meat, poultry, fish, dried peas or beans, lentils, eggs, and nuts). Get 2 to 3 servings per day.

Serving size: A serving of protein consists of 2 to 3 ounces of cooked meat, poultry, or fish; 1 cup of cooked peas, beans, or lentils; two eggs; or 4 tablespoons of peanut butter or about ½ cup of nuts.

Tip: An ounce of meat, poultry, or fish is about the size of a matchbox; 3 ounces is about the size of a deck of cards.

We need protein but not too much. The body uses protein to produce and maintain tissues, manufacture enzymes and hormones, maintain the proper acid-base balance, regulate fluid, and make disease-fighting antibodies. Protein also helps slow the rise of glucose in the bloodstream, thus stabilizing blood sugar levels, so having a small amount of protein with each meal or snack (say, 2 tablespoons of cottage cheese, a slice of cheese, or an ounce of meat, fish, or poultry) can help stave off low blood sugar.

Good sources of protein include lean meats, fish, eggs, poultry, and other foods of animal origin. But you can also get your daily protein in the form of plant foods such as peas, beans, lentils, and certain nuts (specifically peanuts, almonds, and walnuts). Peas, beans, and lentils (all members of the legume family) are especially good for your health because they are rich in vitamins, high in fiber, and low in fat. Because of this, many experts recommend that legumes be eaten at least three times a week.

Dairy (milk, yogurt, and cheese). Get 2 to 3 servings per day.

Serving size: A serving of dairy foods equals 1 cup of milk or yogurt or 1½ to 2 ounces of cheese.

Tip: An ounce of cheese is the size of four dice; a cup of yogurt is the size of a baseball.

The calcium, vitamin D, and protein contributed by dairy foods are all necessary for bone growth and maintenance. Too little calcium in the diet can result in osteoporosis—thinning and hollowing of the bones that can lead to fractures, severe back pain, or spinal deformities.

Fats, oils, and sweets. Use sparingly.

The Food Guide Pyramid's advice to use fats, oils, and sweets sparingly is somewhat enigmatic. Generally, you should use these items in the way you would use condiments—to flavor your foods or add interest to a meal. Many Runaway Eaters consider these foods "bad" and try to avoid them at all costs. But you do need at least 1 serving of fats per day (such as 1 tablespoon of olive oil, butter, trans-free margarine, or mayonnaise) to meet your requirement for essential fatty acids, which play a part in immunity and vision, the formation of cell membranes, and the production of hormonelike compounds, among other things.

Fats in the diet serve a couple of other important purposes as well: They add flavor to food, making it more palatable and enjoyable, and they increase the length of time that you feel satisfied after a meal. Of course, this doesn't mean that you should load up on fatty foods, but it does mean that there's no reason to feel guilty for using a little dressing on your salad or a pat of butter on a slice of whole wheat bread. In fact, it's an excellent idea.

Having a limited amount of sweets may also be a good idea, because this can increase your eating enjoyment and help prevent feelings of deprivation. However, to prevent blood glucose spikes and dips, sweets should be eaten only in small amounts *after* consuming a healthful meal. And, of course, sweets or fats should not be substituted for the health-promoting foods recommended by the Food Guide Pyramid.

Water. Drink eight 8-ounce glasses (½ gallon) per day.

Your body needs at least eight 8-ounce glasses of water every day to replenish lost fluids, wash away toxins, prevent constipation, and reduce water retention or bloating. Sip it a little at a time throughout the day, rather than drinking large amounts all at once. Water is infinitely better for your body than any kind of soft drink—whether the sugary kind or the diet version.

Planning Your Meals

A healthy, balanced meal or snack will contain a grain, a fruit or vegetable, and a protein (or dairy food, because these also contain protein). The grain and fruit or vegetable will give you energy and fiber, and the protein will help stabilize your blood sugar.

What follows is a meal and snack plan that includes the *minimum* number of servings of the food groups that you should eat daily. We've included the size of a typical serving just to give you an idea of how much you need (at the very least) of each kind of food. This is not a diet—it's more of a reality check to remind you that a serving of chicken is neither one bite nor half the bird.

Sample Meal and Snack Plan

Breakfast

     1 serving grains: ½ cup cooked cereal
     ½ serving protein: 1 egg
     ½ serving dairy: ½ cup milk
     1 serving fruits: 1 peach

Lunch

> 2 servings grains: 2 slices whole wheat bread
> 1 serving protein: 2 ounces tuna
> 1 serving vegetables: 1 cup vegetable soup

Snack

> 1 serving grains: 4 whole wheat crackers
> ½ serving dairy: ¾ ounce cheese
> 1 serving vegetables: 1 cup carrot sticks

Dinner

> 2 servings grains: 1 cup pasta
> 1 serving protein: Spaghetti sauce with 2 ounces meat
> 1 serving vegetables: ½ cup cooked zucchini

Snack

> 1 serving grains: 1 slice whole wheat bread
> 1 serving dairy: 1 cup yogurt
> 1 serving fruits: 1 cup sliced strawberries

If you've been restricting for a long period of time, this may seem like too much food. And if you've been bingeing, it may seem like far too little. Consider this meal plan to be a general guide. If you're not getting at least the amounts indicated above of each kind of food, you're shortchanging your health and increasing your risk of Runaway Eating. At a minimum, make sure you're eating the amount of servings indicated at the lower end of the Food Guide Pyramid's recommended ranges.

WHEN TO EAT

Our ancient ancestors ate when food was available and stopped eating when they couldn't hold any more. But today things aren't quite that simple. You're surrounded by food and constantly bombarded with messages to eat. If you ate every time food was available, you'd never stop. To make matters worse, you've probably learned how to ride roughshod over your satiety signals. Even when filled to the bursting point, you may still order a big dessert. Or you may refrain from eating for long hours, or even days, when you're dieting, even though your hunger pangs are booming resoundingly.

Eating to Restore Your Body's Hunger and Satiety Signals

In an ideal world, you'd simply listen to your body's hunger and satiety signals and eat or stop eating on their command. But erratic eating, bingeing, and dieting tend to throw these signals off kilter, so they may no longer be reliable indicators. Your eventual goal is to eat according to your body's signals (as discussed on page 97), but first you'll need to bring them back to normal, which you can do by following the four suggestions below. Before you begin, however, bear in mind that the time it takes for hunger and satiety signals to normalize will vary from person to person. You may find that these signals begin to normalize in a few weeks, or you may find it takes months. Be patient with yourself and stick with the suggestions below. Remember: This is the way your body was designed to work.

Eat regularly and spread out your daily food intake. Feeding your body regularly and well is crucial to overcoming Runaway Eating. Only when your body feels certain that the food supply is plentiful and constant will it be able to relax and stop urging you to overeat.

For our purposes, the definition of *regular eating* is three planned meals plus two or three planned snacks each day, spaced so there is no more than 3 to 4 hours between each one. Meals should be fairly equal in size; make sure you don't overload at any one time. Likewise, keep your snacks about the same size.

In the sample meal and snack plan above, the three regular meals are accompanied by a midafternoon snack to help ward off the energy slump you may feel as the workday winds down, and an evening snack to help fend off urges to binge in the long hours between dinner and breakfast.

You'll notice that we've said "planned" meals and snacks. We recommend that you write down in advance what you're going to eat each day, and make sure you have these foods available, so that there's a minimum of fuss when it's time to eat. This will help you avoid last-minute decisions or emotional eating.

Don't skip breakfast. If you're like a lot of people, breakfast can be a hit-or-miss affair. You might decide to skip it because you just don't feel hungry. Or, if you're rushed in the morning (and who isn't?), you might not want to take the time to eat. Or you might think that skipping breakfast is an easy way to cut back on your calorie intake.

The truth is that skipped or long-delayed meals will set you up for bingeing, and breakfast already qualifies as a long-delayed meal. This makes eating breakfast extra important—in fact, skipping just this one meal can be enough to trigger overeating or bingeing later in the day. Skipping breakfast also lowers your metabolism (making it easier to gain and harder to lose weight) and impairs concentration throughout the morning hours. Although in this book we've tried to stay away from too many "shoulds," the one "should" we feel very strongly about is eating breakfast. So always eat breakfast within about an hour of getting up, and aim to include both protein and carbohydrates to help stabilize your blood sugar and help prolong the feeling of fullness. (The only exception to the protein-and-carb rule concerns Runaway Eaters

IF THE THOUGHT OF A MEAL PLAN MAKES YOU NERVOUS . . .

If you get anxious just by looking at a meal plan or a list of serving sizes, and the Food Guide Pyramid sounds too much like a diet, think about it like this:

- Eat five or six times a day (three meals and two or three snacks).
- Eat at regular intervals, allowing no more than 3 to 4 hours between meals and snacks (except when you're sleeping).
- Try to eat breakfast within 1 hour of arising.
- Aim to include the following combo in meals and snacks: a grain, a protein (or dairy food), and a fruit or vegetable.

who are experiencing problems with depression and may also be struggling with bingeing or anxiety. If this describes you, turn to page 194 for a modified plan.)

Try your best to avoid eating between meals and snacks. Your body needs to learn to tell the difference between having plenty of fuel and running low, and unless you allow 3 to 4 hours of no eating between meals, it can't discover true hunger. Sticking with this on-again, off-again pattern of eating will allow your body's real hunger signals to resurface. If, however, you do end up eating during the off-again period, just continue with your next meal or snack as planned. Don't try to cut back on your food intake to make up for what you've eaten, because this can exacerbate Runaway Eating.

When your body has once again learned to recognize real hunger, you'll be able to eat according to these signals rather than a clock.

Don't get too hung up on measuring. Use the serving sizes as a reference at first. Then, once you can eyeball an average serving size, start thinking more in terms of food groups. (For example, "I need at least some protein, a fruit or vegetable, and a grain for lunch.") Don't weigh and measure every mouthful; this just increases your anxiety levels and encourages both perfectionism and obsessive-compulsive behavior. Too much fussing over getting the exact amount of food can be counterproductive.

HOW TO EAT

How you eat is just as vital to your physical and mental health as what and when you eat. The practices, attitudes, and habits that you bring to the table can do much to discourage Runaway Eating. To beat it for good, you'll want to adopt the following four rules.

- ◆ Give up dieting forever.
- ◆ Eat according to your body's hunger and satiety signals.
- ◆ Give yourself permission to eat.
- ◆ Eat foods you really enjoy.

Rule I: Give Up Dieting Forever

It's vital that you give up the idea and the practice of dieting— permanently. By *dieting* we mean restricting calories below a healthy level in order to lose weight, restricting yourself to certain kinds or combinations of food, or doing both. Restricting in either of these ways can trigger binges, slow your metabolism, encourage obsessive eating behaviors, and interfere with your body's natural hunger and satiety signals. Diets, in general, can also lower serotonin levels, and low serotonin has been linked to depression, anxiety, bingeing, and a craving for sweets. (No wonder diets make most people want to eat more than ever before!) This effect may be especially problematic with low-carbohydrate diets. Studies have shown that potential production of serotonin in healthy women can drop after they've dieted for as few as 3 weeks. Animal studies have also shown that food restriction lowers both levels of serotonin and its rate of production in the brain.

Still giving up dieting can be easier said than done. There is a certain amount of security found in following set guidelines and dictums. Dieters often feel relieved that the diet frees them from the responsibility of choosing their own kinds and amounts of food. So without the structure of a diet, longtime dieters can feel lost and afraid. Because of this, many former dieters cling to dieting principles even when they think they've given up the practice. Unconsciously, they find ways to restrict their food intake and keep themselves on track. We call this the dieting mindset. Unfortunately, the dieting mindset is just as destructive as dieting itself and does much to keep Runaway Eating behaviors alive and well. To determine if this could be a problem for you, take the "Do You Have the Dieting Mindset?" quiz on page 98. In the following chapters, we'll share proven strategies to overcome this mindset, by recognizing and changing destructive thought patterns and transforming negative moods without the use of food.

Rule 2: Eat According to Your Body's Hunger and Satiety Signals

After you've been eating regular meals and snacks according to the suggestions in the "When to Eat" section, your hunger and satiety signals should begin to become more reliable indicators of when and how much your body needs to eat. When you feel comfortable, you'll want to begin to respond to these signals—eating when you feel hungry and terminating a meal or snack as soon

DO YOU HAVE THE DIETING MINDSET?

Even long after they've given up dieting, many people still retain
the dieting mindset. This destructive way of thinking can hinder your
recovery from Runaway Eating, because it impairs your ability to recognize your body's hunger and satiety signals. To see if you're still
combating the dieting mindset, answer "true" or "false" to the
following statements.

__ 1. There are certain foods that I consider "good" and certain foods
       I consider "bad."

__ 2. I mentally tally up the number of calories I eat each day to keep
       from overdoing it.

__ 3. I always weigh and measure my food before eating.

__ 4. I'm never hungry for breakfast, so I don't waste the calories on it.

__ 5. One of my goals is to fit into a too-small dress, skirt, or pair of
       pants that is hanging in my closet.

__ 6. I try to go as long as possible before eating.

__ 7. I think about food almost all the time.

__ 8. There are things I'd like to eat, but I avoid them because I'd never
       stop eating them once I got started.

__ 9. I avoid carbs.

__ 10. I drink a lot of coffee, tea, or diet soft drinks to try to fill up so I'll
       eat less.

If you answered "true" to any of these questions, you may still be dieting, even though you think you aren't. Make a conscious effort to stop
restricting the overall amount and the kinds of food you eat. The more
you restrict, the more likely you are to binge.

as you feel full. To help you do this, try the Recognizing Your Hunger Technique. While continuing with your eating plan, do the following:

- Listen for the signs of hunger—a growling in your stomach, perhaps a feeling of light-headedness or being slightly weak, or an increase in saliva production. The signals may be weak, so heighten your awareness.

- As soon as you feel the slightest sense of hunger, eat a healthy snack. It doesn't matter what time it is or how long it's been since you last ate. When your body says it's time to eat, feed it. (This contradicts our earlier suggestion that you refrain from eating between meals and snacks. It's all right in this case because you're trying out a new technique.)

- Once you've eaten your snack, relax and notice how your body feels now that its hunger signals have been recognized. (It may take up to 20 minutes before you feel the changes, because the signals have to travel from your stomach to your brain.)

- Continue to eat your meals and snacks according to schedule, but delay them up to 30 minutes if you don't yet feel hungry. If hunger doesn't surface after a 30-minute delay, go ahead and eat the meal or snack anyway.

- When you do have a meal or snack, eat slowly and listen to your body's cues. The minute you get the feeling of fullness, stop eating and sit with the feeling for a few minutes. If it goes away and you feel like eating more, go ahead. If you still feel full, stop eating, put the food away, and leave the table. Remind yourself that you can come back and eat more whenever you feel hungry, but don't continue to eat once you feel full.

This is slightly different from the way you were eating when you were trying to normalize your body's signals. That's because after you have gotten used to eating standard amounts of food on a regular schedule, you need to learn to let your body tell you when and how much to eat. But this will work only if you are eating solely in response to sensations of physical hunger. If you're eating be-

DON'T LET RESTAURANTS DICTATE YOUR PORTION SIZE

Okay, so you've given yourself permission to eat, and you're trying to tune in to your body's hunger and satiety signals. But then you go out to eat and are faced with mammoth portions of food that by their mere presence can make you want to binge. Served on platters instead of plates, some of these offerings could easily feed an entire family. For example, it's not uncommon for a restaurant to serve a 16-ounce steak, even though 1 serving of protein is just 2 to 3 ounces, or the size of a deck of cards.

At times like these, it's hard to rely on body cues alone to help you determine how much you

need to eat. To help yourself, try drawing a line down the center of your plate with your knife and cutting off the portion sizes that you think are accurate. Put them to one side (the "I am going to eat" side), while the remainder stays on the "doggy bag" side. This makes it clear from the beginning that the restaurant does not dictate how much you should eat. If you worry that you'll still be tempted to clean your plate, ask for a doggy bag even before you take your first bite. That way, you'll have an appropriate portion size on your plate, and the rest will be packed away out of sight for tomorrow's dinner.

cause of boredom, depression, nervousness, or any other cause, then you aren't tuning in to your hunger and satiety signals. In fact, you're actually promoting Runaway Eating.

Rule 3: Give Yourself Permission to Eat

Giving yourself permission to eat might be the single scariest thing you need to do to recover from Runaway Eating. You may think that if you just let go and eat, you'll never stop. Actually, the reverse is true. Abnormally restricting your food can make you want to eat insatiably. Once you begin eating regularly, your desire to binge will recede and maybe even vanish completely.

You may be afraid that your weight will skyrocket when you start eating regularly, but studies show that this isn't usually the case as long as your portion sizes are sensible. Your weight will most likely either stay the same or decrease, mostly because you'll no longer be overeating or bingeing. And once you add in reasonable amounts of physical activity, your weight should normalize.

Rule 4: Eat Foods You Really Enjoy

In the race to become skinny, healthy, or gorgeous (or all three), we often forget that eating should be one of life's most pleasurable and satisfying experiences. How often have you remarked that everything that tastes good is bad for you? Or that everything that's good for you is tasteless?

Foods that taste good can also be good for you, and you don't have to give up the foods you love in order to be healthy and attractive. In fact, avoiding your favorite foods may be exactly the wrong thing to do, since this encourages bingeing and

ENJOYABLE EATING DO'S AND DON'TS

Enjoyable Eating can do a lot to lower diet-related anxiety and depression, increase self-confidence, decrease perfectionism, and improve your relationship with food. It may even result in weight loss as you leave bingeing and overeating behind, although this shouldn't be your primary goal. But like everything else, Enjoyable Eating has certain guidelines that need to be respected.

Do's

- Do eat what you really want, but make it a part of a generally healthy, balanced eating plan. (Don't live on just one or two kinds of food.)
- Do prepare tasty, attractive, appealing meals and snacks for yourself.
- Do honor the principles of good nutrition as much as possible, without pressuring yourself to consume the world's healthiest diet.
- Do take time out, sit down, and really pay attention to your food while you're eating, whether it's a meal or a snack.
- Do slow down. It takes less food to gain the same amount of satisfaction when you cut it up, eat it at a leisurely pace, and relax while eating.
- Do really taste your food, chew it slowly, and get as much enjoyment as you can out of every bite.
- Do eat in response to hunger

preoccupation with food and makes you feel deprived. Eventually, eating these forbidden foods (which most of us do) contributes to a sense of failure and lowers self-esteem.

Instead, we suggest that you practice what we call Enjoyable Eating. That is, eat the foods you love, but in reasonable amounts. Choose foods that are good for your tastebuds *and* your health. Do you like macaroni and cheese? Frozen yogurt? Teriyaki steak? In moderation, these can all be considered foods that contribute

and stop as soon as you feel full, as often as possible.

Don'ts

- Don't label foods as "good" or "bad." All foods can be a part of a health-promoting, satisfying diet, as long as you don't overdo it in any one area. Calling a food "bad" makes it more alluring and can trigger bingeing.
- Don't take the focus off your food by watching TV, reading, driving, or doing computer work while eating.
- Don't eat while standing over the sink, in front of the refrigerator, or while cooking.
- Don't sacrifice healthy, regular eating in order to eat according to your hunger and satiety signals before they normalize. That is, if you feel hungry every 5 minutes, don't act on it. Conversely, if you don't feel hungry until 3:00 in the afternoon, eat your regular meals and snacks at the proper time anyway.
- Don't compensate for overeating or bingeing by skipping meals, eating less, purging, exercising excessively, or taking laxatives or diuretics. This will just keep you on the Runaway Eating merry-go-round indefinitely.
- Don't eat in response to your emotions.
- Don't use alcohol or recreational drugs. These substances undermine your self-control and alter your perception.

to good health. Try eating a standard serving size of a favorite food as part of one of your regular meals or snacks. At the end of the day, think about how you felt about eating this food, how it tasted, and what you did after you ate it. Did it make you want to binge? Did you feel better or worse? Did it add to your enjoyment, or did it increase your stress levels? You may find that you can eat standard amounts of many of the foods that you love without experiencing any adverse consequences. And because you don't give these foods special power, and your stress levels don't skyrocket because you're trying so hard to avoid them, they are not nearly as likely to trigger Runaway Eating as they used to be.

There may be foods, however, that make you feel worse by triggering binges, anxiety, or excessive stress. If you find it difficult to add enjoyable foods to your food plan, or there are a number of foods you'd like to eat that are problematic for you, consider seeing a registered dietitian who specializes in the treatment of eating disorders and can help you slowly integrate these foods into a healthful diet.

CHAPTER 6

Identify Your Triggers

No matter what form your Runaway Eating takes, it will never do what it's "supposed" to do. You may stuff yourself in order to feel better, diet rigorously to get thin, or exercise excessively or purge to gain control of your body. But inevitably, all of these strategies will fail. You don't feel better, you don't get thin, and you don't control your urges. Yet, like tens of thousands of other women, you can find yourself caught in a never-ending cycle of these seemingly pointless behaviors. Why? Because in spite of its obvious connection to food, *Runaway Eating is not about food, diets, or weight loss.* Instead, it serves a very specific function in your life. It's an attempt to meet certain needs that aren't being met in other ways, to deal with or defend against whatever has become unmanageable.

Runaway Eating offers short-term, immediate "solutions" that have no positive long-term effects. Certainly, it's not the bingeing, starving, or purging that attracts someone to Runaway Eating. It's the emotional benefits that these behaviors bring about. So before you can change your Runaway Eating behaviors, you need to discover what functions these behaviors serve in your life and why.

WHAT'S THE POINT OF RUNAWAY EATING?

When you don't feel good about yourself or your life, it's natural to try to do something to rectify things. Runaway Eating is an attempt to turn wrongs into rights, to change bad feelings to good ones. It may temporarily distract you, ease your anxiety, assuage your fears, help you express certain inexpressible feelings, or make you feel that you're in control. Although it won't solve these problems, it does serve as a kind of bandage that can hide the pain and the terrible feelings—for a while.

Thinking about the form that your Runaway Eating takes—whether it's bingeing, purging, or restrictive eating—may help you to define its purpose in your life.

What Functions Are Served by Bingeing?

Binge-eating is a classic way to stuff down painful emotions, especially for those who shrink from confrontation or have trouble putting their feelings into words. If you binge, you may be seeking:

Relief from tension. Anxiety levels are often high in those with problematic eating, particularly if they've been dieting, and one way to get relief is simply to let go and eat.

Comfort, soothing, consolation. If you've ever eaten a box of candy when you were feeling down, you know that food can have a comforting, sedating effect (particularly if it's high in carbohydrates). Food is the original source of instant gratification, a way to make yourself feel better *now.*

Distraction, numbness, and escape from unwanted experiences. It's so much easier to bury yourself in a gallon of ice cream than to confront problems head-on or feel unpleasant emotions. Some women who binge will talk about going into a "binge mode" while eating, during which they feel nothing, their eyes glaze over, and all thoughts and feelings are temporarily placed on hold.

Avoidance of intimacy. If you fear intimacy, have experienced sexual abuse or assault in the past, or want to distance yourself from sexuality, gaining weight through bingeing may be your way of armoring yourself and discouraging sexual advances.

What Functions Are Served by Purging?

After bingeing, some Runaway Eaters feel intensely guilty and anxious and may try to compensate for their actions by inducing vomiting, abusing laxatives or diuretics, or exercising excessively. If you purge, you may be seeking:

Relief from guilt, fear, and anxiety. Although ineffective as a weight-control method, purging is an instant way to relieve the intense guilt, fear, and anxiety that follow a binge. But precisely because purging gives you an out, it helps to keep the binge cycle going.

Self-punishment. Inducing vomiting, exercising to the point of exhaustion, or taking laxatives is the price some Runaway Eaters extract from themselves for falling off their diets. In fact, the more unpleasant the punishment, the more relief they may feel.

An outlet for anger. Many Runaway Eaters have a great deal of trouble expressing anger directly. Some find that the only way they can exorcise their anger demons is by purging.

A high. The act of purging can trigger the release of certain chemicals in the brain that bring about feelings of relaxation, relief, and well-being. This may be the body's way of compensating

THE CONSEQUENCES OF RUNAWAY EATING: THE GOOD, THE BAD, AND THE UGLY

For every short-term positive function served by Runaway Eating, there is a long-term negative consequence. Consider the following:

Short-Term Function	Long-Term Result
Avoidance of conflict (bingeing, purging, restricting, exercising)	Isolation, detachment, withdrawal from others, lying, decreased trust in relationships
Avoidance of tasks deemed overwhelming (bingeing, purging, restricting, exercising)	Problems performing at work and home, procrastination, lack of focus, important tasks left undone
Reduced hunger (bingeing)	Increased risk of obesity, heart disease, diabetes, arthritis, depression, acid reflux
Comfort, consolation (bingeing)	Depression, disgust, self-deprecation
Emotional anesthesia; temporary relief of anger, guilt, tension, boredom, frustration, anxiety, fear (bingeing, purging, restricting, exercising)	Depression, shame, guilt, hopelessness, feeling worthless and out of control
Temporary reduction in worries or unpleasant thoughts (bingeing, purging, restricting, exercising)	Increase in feelings of being out of control, decrease in self-esteem
Feelings of being in control, self-punishment to maintain discipline and control (purging, restricting, exercising)	Depression, lack of control, anxiety about ability to maintain controlling behaviors
A way to "prove yourself" (restricting, exercising)	Increased anxiety, feeling that it doesn't prove anything
Avoidance of intimacy (bingeing, purging, restricting, exercising)	Lack of satisfying relationships, loneliness, isolation

for the violence it experiences during purging; it blocks the pain and promotes a high feeling. Those who purge can become dependent on this high, and some will purge even when they haven't binged, just to experience the physiological rush.

What Functions Are Served by Restrictive Eating?

For some, restrictive eating provides structure, control, or a way to prove mastery over their minds and bodies. If you restrict your eating, you may be seeking:

Structure, consistency, control. If everything else in your life feels out of your control, your diet may be the one thing that's clear cut and concrete. It's all good or bad, right or wrong, allowable or forbidden.

A way to prove yourself worthy. Fasting or rigid dieting involves a denial of self that saints and religious martyrs have used for centuries to purify themselves and prove their worthiness. If you're a restricting type of Runaway Eater, you may employ these same techniques to bolster your flagging self-esteem.

A means of numbing anxiety or unpleasant moods. In some people, restrictive eating actually *decreases* anxiety, irritability, and unpleasant moods—exactly the opposite of the reactions it promotes in most people. Some restricting Runaway Eaters may use dieting and fasting to ease an all-pervasive sense of anxiety or doom and gloom.

HOW THOUGHTS AND FEELINGS LEAD TO BEHAVIORS

As you can see, although food and weight obsessions may seem to be about the body, they are really about what's going on in your mind. Your habitual thoughts—especially those that aren't true—play an important role in shaping your self-image and can contribute to distorted ideas about yourself, weight, food, and the world around you. These distorted ideas, in turn, lead you to develop negative feelings about yourself, which prompt unhealthy compensatory behaviors, such as Runaway Eating.

Thought Myths

Your thoughts are a kind of running commentary on yourself and the world around you. You may not even be aware of many of them until you tune in and really pay attention. Some of your thoughts may have no basis in fact, but you've probably accepted them without question. We call these Thought Myths, because they arise from faulty logic and invalid statements.

Thought Myths concerning yourself define who and what you think you are and can be prime contributors to Runaway Eating. They can include statements like:

- "I can't control myself around food."
- "I have no willpower."
- "I've always been fat, and I'll always be fat."
- "If I eat foods that contain sugar, I totally lose control."
- "I can't be beautiful unless I'm thin."
- "Being overweight is a sign that I'm lazy."

Thought Myths like these pave the way to low self-esteem, destructive self-fulfilling prophecies, and unhealthy ways of coping. In chapter 7, we'll discuss how to replace these Thought Myths with healthy, accurate thoughts.

Feelings: How Does It Feel to Be You?

Feelings, or emotions, can be much harder to identify than thoughts. Although thoughts can usually be defined in sentences or images, feelings can be difficult to express in words or pictures. Sometimes you may not know how you feel. Feelings also differ from thoughts because they come in varying intensities. You may feel slightly angry, exceedingly happy, or somewhat excited.

Your thoughts, whether accurate or mythical, affect your feelings. For example, let's say that you just tried on a bathing suit and you don't like the way you look. If you think to yourself, "I'm a disgusting, fat pig! I'll never look right in a bathing suit," you'll probably feel worthless, depressed, and ready to binge or starve. But if you think, "This bathing suit isn't right for me. I need to find one that's more flattering to my figure," you may feel better about yourself.

Your thoughts and feelings affect each other interchangeably. A thought may prompt a feeling (thinking "I need to exercise" may make you feel anxious if you're short on time), and a feeling may prompt a thought (a lingering feeling of sadness may lead to thoughts of eating potato chips).

Behaviors: The Product of Thoughts and Feelings

Like dominoes, your thoughts and feelings lead to behaviors, or the things that you do. Runaway Eating is almost always the product of Thought Myths concerning your relationship with food or your beliefs about weight, plus negative feelings about yourself. Imagine the following scenario: Janet's boss sends her an e-mail saying that he'd like to see her at 3:00 P.M. for an im-promptu meeting. The way Janet chooses to think about this e-mail will make all the difference in the way she behaves.

Example 1: After Janet gets the e-mail, she thinks:

Thought: "Uh oh, here we go. I've done a lousy job, and he's going to fire me; I just know it!"

Feelings: Janet is panicky, tense, worried, and very upset. She feels an impending sense of doom and wants to disappear, escape, run out of the office.

Behavior: Overcome with anxiety, she hurries to the company cafeteria and buys an ice cream bar, a couple of candy bars, and a piece of cake. She stuffs it all down while standing outside behind the building, where no one will see her. She doesn't really feel any better, but she just can't seem to stop herself.

On the other hand, when Janet thinks about the situation in a healthier, more positive way, her behavior changes completely.

Example 2: After Janet gets the e-mail, she thinks:

Thought: "Well, I've certainly tried my best. He'll probably give me a good evaluation."

Feelings: Janet is calm and in control. Although she's curious about the meeting, she anticipates a positive result.

Behavior: She continues with her work until 3:00 P.M., then confidently walks into her boss's office for her meeting.

Clearly, just by changing a single thought, Janet could channel her feelings and behavior in either direction, positive or negative.

The good news is that you can do the same. By learning simple techniques for changing your thoughts, you can start to reestablish a healthy relationship with food and your own body. The fancy name for these techniques is cognitive-behavioral therapy, but the important thing to remember is that they'll help you reclaim control over your thoughts, feelings, and—ultimately—your Runaway Eating behavior. And the first step in regaining that control is to identify the cues that start the process.

CUES: WHAT SETS IT ALL OFF

A cue is anything that triggers an unhealthy thought or feeling that leads to a Runaway Eating behavior. In the example above, the e-mail from Janet's boss was a cue for her.

Generally, the cues that trigger Runaway Eating fall into one of the six categories described below. These categories aren't mutually exclusive, however; many cues will fall into more than one category.

Social cues. Food and social events go hand in hand, and being around people (or feeling isolated from them) can be a strong cue for triggering Runaway Eating. Sometimes eating behaviors are used to avoid interpersonal conflict, such as eating rather than having a fight with your partner, or to assuage fears of an upcoming event, such as speaking in public or going on a date.

Food cues. Just being around chocolate cake, fried chicken, or other high-risk foods may be enough to set you off. Other food cues include going to the grocery store, passing a fast-food restaurant or bakery, looking at food advertisements, and going out to eat. Drinking alcohol can bring on Runaway Eating primarily because it lowers inhibitions.

(continued on page 116)

CONTROLLING THE CUES

Because cues trip the switch that sets Runaway Eating in motion, it makes sense to try to become aware of your cues and do what you can to keep them in check. Consider these strategies.

Be prepared. Do what you can to defuse high-risk setups for Runaway Eating. For example, if you know that you usually binge as soon as you get home from work, have a light snack before you leave work, or have a healthful snack or meal waiting for you in the refrigerator so that you can sit down and eat immediately. When you're finished, take a bath or a walk—anything that will get you out of the kitchen before you start to binge.

Avoid the impossible whenever possible. What's your Achilles' heel: All-you-can-eat buffets? Nerve-wracking cocktail parties? Walking by the vending machines at work? Avoid these cues, if possible. Stay away from the buffets, beg off from the cocktail parties, and take a different route so that you don't need to pass the vending machines. You may learn to handle these cues eventually, but right now it's a good idea to steer clear.

When you eat, just eat. Do you watch TV, drive, read, work, or cook while eating? Combining eating with other activities can cause you to lose touch with your body's hunger and satiety signals and increase the tendency to binge. Make a point of sitting down and focusing only on your food and, perhaps, on the company of others. You'll eat less in the long run and enjoy your food more.

Forget about food when it's not mealtime. Many Runaway Eaters think about food all day long, no matter what they're doing (a common side effect of dieting). To avoid this, make sure you always eat regular, satisfying meals and snacks. And during times when boredom usually sets in, do your best to keep your mind active, get engrossed in a hobby, or keep your hands busy by doing woodwork, knitting, or making crafts. If you have spare time, you might think about volunteering to help others who have more problems than you do—it's a great way to take your mind off yourself.

Build up your healthy cues. Put your running shoes by the door so that you can pull them on for a quick predinner walk. Chop vegetables for a stir-fry and put them up front in the refrigerator so that you won't have an excuse not to cook. Take a bath during the late-night hour when you would normally head for the ice cream. Cues trigger healthy behavior just as surely as they trigger unhealthy behavior. Figure out which ones will work for you, and then use them.

Wait a minute! When you feel the urge to engage in Runaway Eating behaviors, pause before reacting for, say, 5 minutes. The idea is to take back at least some control of the situation. (Yes, you binged, but you waited a full 5 minutes before doing so. That means your Runaway Eating didn't run away with you completely.)

Then next time it happens, increase the pause to 10 minutes and try rerouting your thoughts to come up with a healthier behavior. (See chapter 7.)

Do something different. When you feel that a Runaway Eating episode is about to overtake you, remove yourself from the scene and go do something else. Get out of the kitchen, leave the restaurant, walk away from the food court, get off the exercise bike, get out of the bathroom. Take a walk, go for a drive, get a massage, get your nails done, do some gardening, call a friend. Take the energy you'd normally channel into Runaway Eating and apply it in a healthier, more positive way.

Pat yourself on the back. Praise yourself for every single victory, no matter how small. For example, if you put off bingeing for 5 minutes, tell yourself, "That was great. I'm learning control." Or if you ate a good breakfast even though you binged the night before, applaud yourself for starting the day in a healthy way.

Body cues. Being hungry, feeling tired, being premenstrual, or going through perimenopause or menopause can make you feel like eating anything and everything. Even feeling full can be a body cue for bingeing, by prompting thoughts like "I've already blown it, so I might as well eat some more."

Thought cues. If you're running old movies in your head that feature fights with your loved ones, sexual abuse, or other negative memories of the past, you may be setting yourself up for a bout of Runaway Eating. Thoughts of the future can have a similar effect, particularly if you're anxious about upcoming events. On a completely different note, you may think that you deserve to eat whatever you want because you've been "good" for a certain amount of time.

Feeling cues. Feelings, whether happy or sad, often trigger Runaway Eating behaviors, which act as a kind of emotional anesthesia. The most common feeling cues include depression, boredom, anxiety, elation, excitement, anger, frustration, guilt, and shame.

Environmental cues. Sometimes cues pop up when you least expect them. Going to the movies and admiring the super-slim female lead, being around an attractive friend, listening to others talk about food or eating, or going shopping for clothes may be enough to get the Runaway Eating ball rolling.

Determining the cues that trigger your bouts of Runaway Eating is the first step to ending the cycle. Make a list of all the things you can think of that set off your Runaway Eating behavior. Try to include at least one cue from each of the categories above. For example, Dee, a 45-year-old massage therapist, listed the following as her cues for Runaway Eating: fast-food places, being alone, work-related tension, fatigue, fights with her husband, worrying about getting old, boredom, and going to all-you-can-eat buffets.

You may be surprised at how many different things can set you up for Runaway Eating.

WHAT'S SETTING YOU OFF?

Now that you understand how Runaway Eating develops, it's time to take a closer look at the cues, thoughts, and feelings that are triggering your problem. In order to do this, you'll need to self-monitor, which means recording every day what you eat and the situations, thoughts, and feelings that accompany your eating. It's best to do this right after you eat each meal or snack so that you can really tune in to the thoughts and feelings you were experiencing at the time. The purpose is not to make you focus on every bite you take or analyze what you are or aren't eating; it's to understand the patterns behind your eating behaviors and discover what triggers the unhealthy ones.

How to Self-Monitor

The key to successful self-monitoring is doing it every day. We recommend that you start with a week and include a weekend, because that's when most people eat differently (usually more). Photocopy the blank sheet on page 118, or write out the column heads in a journal or notebook. Then record the following information.

- Time: Note the time of day you ate or drank something.
- Food, drink, and amount: Write down everything you ate or drank at that time, even if it was just a couple of chips or a sip of milk.
- B/P/R/C: This stands for "binge," "purge," "restrict," and

DAILY LOG FOR SELF-MONITORING

DATE: _____

Time	Food, Drink, and Amount	B/P/R/C	Situation/Place	Thoughts	Feelings	Intensity (0–10)

"crave." If you think you've engaged in any of these behaviors, or you had a strong urge to do so (a craving), put down the appropriate code.

- Situation/Place: Jot down where you were, who you were with, and a brief description of what was happening around you at the time.
- Thoughts: Record what you were thinking about before and during eating. These don't have to be thoughts related to food. In fact, you should look beyond food thoughts to figure out what other kinds of thoughts may be contributing to your Runaway Eating.
- Feelings: Note how you felt before and during eating. These should not be feelings related to food. What else was going on with your feelings at that moment?
- Intensity: Rate the strength of these feelings on a scale of 0 to 10, with 0 being no feelings at all and 10 being extremely intense feelings.

Analyzing Your Daily Log for Self-Monitoring

Once you've filled out a week's worth of logs, look over them and answer these questions.

1. What times of the day did you typically engage in unhealthy eating behaviors?

What to look for: Try to identify your high-risk times. Did you tend to binge in the late afternoon? Did you restrict in the mornings? Did your purging happen mostly after dinner?

What to aim for: Plan ahead to help deal with the urges by scheduling activities during your high-risk times: Go to yoga class, take a hot bath, or call your best friend.

2. Did you eat breakfast every day?

What to look for: On days that you skipped breakfast, chances are you engaged in at least some Runaway Eating behaviors (most likely bingeing).

What to aim for: Make sure that you eat breakfast every day and that it includes protein (for example, an egg, a piece of cheese, or some cottage cheese) to help keep your blood sugar on an even keel and prolong feelings of fullness. (The only exception to this rule concerns Runaway Eaters who are experiencing problems with depression and may also be struggling with bingeing or anxiety. If this describes you, turn to page 194 for a modified plan.) Eating a healthful breakfast is one of the best ways to prevent bingeing later in the day.

3. Did you eat enough and often enough?

What to look for: You should be getting three meals and two or three snacks every day. If you ate less than this, you were restricting.

What to aim for: Eat regular meals and snacks in at least the amounts recommended in chapter 5.

4. Where did you engage in most of your unhealthy eating behaviors?

What to look for: Did they usually occur in your kitchen, in front of your TV, in your bed, in your bathroom, at your in-laws' house, at the mall, or in your car? Look for a pattern.

What to aim for: Now that you know your high-risk places, avoid them, if possible, or designate them as "no food" or "no restrict" zones, depending upon your problem. Later, you'll learn how to face high-risk places head-on.

5. Were there any particular people who seemed to be associated with your unhealthy eating behaviors?

What to look for: Was there someone who always seemed to

be around (or on your mind) when you engaged in an unhealthy eating behavior? Again, look for a pattern.

What to aim for: Sometimes a particular person can be a powerful cue for your unhealthy eating behavior. If this is the case, try to stay away from that person when it's time to eat. Before and during all your dealings with this person, remind yourself that this is a high-risk time. Stay alert and on top of your urges.

6. Which thoughts seemed to be associated with your unhealthy eating behaviors?

What to look for: Did you binge, purge, or restrict because of Thought Myths like "I can't control myself" or "Losing weight is the answer to all my problems"? Look for patterns in your thinking that seem to lead to Runaway Eating.

What to aim for: Once you've identified your Thought Myths, debunk them and replace them with healthier thoughts. (We'll discuss how in chapter 7.)

7. Which feelings seemed to be associated with your unhealthy eating behaviors?

What to look for: How were you feeling before and during episodes of unhealthy eating? Were you bored? Anxious? Sad? These are probably strong cues for your Runaway Eating.

What to aim for: Once you understand which feelings are cues, you can use these feelings as warning signs of an upcoming episode. See chapter 7 for tips on dealing with feelings that lead to episodes of Runaway Eating.

8. Did your feelings tend to run either very high on the emotional intensity scale (ratings 7 to 10), or very low (0 to 2)? Or did you bounce from high to low and back again?

What to look for: Ratings of 7 or higher mean that you tended to set yourself up for emotional burnout. Ratings of 0 to 2 mean that you either were not feeling much at all or were suppressing the feelings you did have. And if your emotions ran from low to high and back again, you're probably on an emotional roller coaster. Any of these emotional states can inflame unhealthy eating behaviors.

What to aim for: The goal is to achieve emotional balance—which is a lot easier said than done. If you're having emotional problems or feel that your emotions have somehow become un-balanced, see chapters 7, 9, 10, and 12 for help in easing anxiety, depression, and the tension caused by perfectionism.

9. Was your eating on the weekend different from your eating during the week?

What to look for: What was your weekend eating pattern? Eating fewer but larger meals, frequent snacking or general grazing, drinking more alcohol? All of these are common because of greater amounts of unstructured time and more family activi-ties and socializing.

What to aim for: Whether it's a weekend or a weekday, try to maintain a predictable eating pattern. Eat about the same amount of food at approximately the same time of day, so your body won't have to adjust to erratic mealtimes or unusually small or large meals.

———— ∞◊∞ ————

By keeping up with your "Daily Logs for Self-Monitoring," you can keep in touch with what's going on inside—physically, men-tally, and emotionally—and plan successful strategies to ward off future bouts of Runaway Eating.

CHAPTER 7

Reroute Your Thinking

E verything would fall into place in my life if only I could get thin."

"If I eat even one bite of cake, I'll lose control and eat the entire thing."

"If I can just lose 15 pounds, my husband will love me more."

Do any of these thoughts sound familiar? Thoughts like these lie at the root of almost all Runaway Eating and may be so much a part of your habitual thinking that you aren't even aware of them.

If you're a Runaway Eater, food, food-related behaviors, or weight may have taken on special, unwarranted powers for you. You may believe that you're literally unable to resist the temptation of a chocolate cake, or you may be convinced that reaching a certain weight goal will make your marriage happier or your friends like you better. Of course, such thoughts are not only untrue but also downright unhealthy. The key to recovery from Runaway Eating lies in using simple strategies—known as cognitive-behavioral skills—to tune in to your thoughts, challenge your Thought Myths, and replace them with healthy, rational thoughts. Continuing to think the same destructive thoughts is like going down the same old roads to the same old destinations. But when you reroute those negative thoughts, you will be traveling new avenues that will get you off the Runaway Highway for good.

KINDS OF THOUGHT MYTHS

Runaway Eaters often have certain ideas about food, weight, themselves, and the world around them that are fundamentally incorrect. Read through the following and see which ones sound familiar to you.

The Thinness Myth

Motto:　"Thinness equals happiness and success."

Rationale: Those who are thin are happier, more attractive, more successful, and richer than those who aren't. (This idea is perpetuated by the media.)

The truth: Happiness is dependent on a lot of different things: satisfying relationships, good health, a sense of purpose, security, and leisure, to name a few. Being thin may make you feel better about yourself, but it does little to enhance these other factors.

The Need for Distraction or Comfort

Motto:　"If I eat enough cookies, I'll feel better."

Rationale: Eating helps you tune out the world, block unpleasant feelings, and fill up emotional emptiness through the sensual pleasures offered by food.

The truth: Food or food-related behaviors are poor substitutes for dealing with the troubles they mask. They just distract you, keep you from getting to the root of your problems, and can cause additional problems such as guilt or low self-esteem.

All-or-Nothing Thinking

Motto: "Either I'm thin or I'm fat. Either I'm good or I'm bad. Either I'm perfect or I'm a failure."

Rationale: Everything is clear cut and neatly laid out: Either it's right or it's wrong. There's no gray area, nothing to wonder about, no hedging.

The truth: There are many shades of gray between black and white, and many possible solutions to a problem. Because people are rarely perfect, all-or-nothing thinking provides an ideal setup for failure. All tasks become impossible when you think this way.

The Need to Be Unique

Motto: "Successful dieting is what sets me apart from everyone else."

Rationale: Pursuing a difficult goal, following strict rules, and behaving in a certain way makes you special, unique, and worthy of attention.

The truth: The symptoms of Runaway Eating can become such a part of your identity that, without them, you may not know who you are or why anyone would pay attention to you.

The Need to Be in Control

Motto: "If I can control my eating, I can control my life."

Rationale: Your life may be chaotic and crazy, and you think you can't do anything about that. But you can do something about your eating.

The truth: Runaway Eating behaviors may make you feel as if you're in control and powerful. In reality, these behaviors control you.

The Need for Instant Gratification

Motto: "I have to make myself feel better now. I can't wait another minute."

Rationale: Food can alter your emotional state in a matter of seconds. One bite of chocolate can instantly relax you and make you happy.

The truth: Food may bring about some short-term emotional benefits, but it does nothing in the long term. Eating for emotional reasons undermines your problem-solving skills and can lead to weight gain, bloating, bingeing, purging, and the resultant depression, guilt, disgust, and self-hatred.

The Need to Be Perfect

Motto: "Anything less than perfection is worthless."

Rationale: If you are the best at everything, work hard enough, don't make any mistakes, and can please everyone, then and only then will you be worthwhile.

The truth: This is the impossible dream. If this is what you are striving for, you will fail.

Magical Thinking

Motto: "Losing weight will radically change my life."

Rationale: All your problems stem from one thing (too much weight). Once you fix it, everything else will fall in line, and you'll be happy and content.

The truth: Your problems (like everyone else's) are many and varied. Solving one problem will change only the things directly related to it. (For example, losing weight may lower your blood pressure and allow you to wear a smaller dress size, but it will not automati-

cally make your children proud of you or improve
your financial situation.)

Overgeneralizing

Motto: "I binged last night; I'll never be able to control my
eating."

Rationale: If you do one thing wrong, you condemn yourself as
a person. If one thing turns out badly, then everything will turn out badly.

The truth: You're drawing broad conclusions based on an isolated incident. The outcome of a single event doesn't
determine the outcome of a group of events. Think of
the World Series.

Catastrophizing

Motto: "I ate an entire quart of ice cream by myself. I can
never be trusted around food again."

Rationale: If one thing goes wrong, it's a disaster. You may as
well just give up.

The truth: This kind of thinking involves a combination of perfectionism and overgeneralizing. No one is perfect,
and no one mistake can doom the overall cause.

Personal Ineffectiveness

Motto: "I know I should eat breakfast, but I just can't make
myself do it."

Rationale: You may be weak, and there are a lot of things that are
too hard for you to do. You'd rather give up than try.

The truth: You're capable of more than you think. Make an
effort and then pat yourself on the back when you
succeed.

WHAT ARE YOUR THOUGHT MYTHS?

To alter your behavior, you must change your thoughts. And to change your thoughts, you must first become aware of them. You do this by really listening and tuning in to what you're thinking, particularly during high-risk times, like when you're trying on clothes or weighing yourself. If you've been diligent about filling in your "Daily Logs for Self-Monitoring" from chapter 6, you've probably found that they're full of clues as to the kinds of Thought Myths that power your Runaway Eating.

Using the descriptions and examples of Thought Myths, plus the information from your daily logs, make a list of your own Thought Myths. (Hint: Thought Myths often make you feel anxious, depressed, guilty, angry, or hopeless.)

By writing down your Thought Myths, you will already be on the way to developing healthier thinking and behavior. Once you're aware of some of your Thought Myths, you can be on the lookout for them. They will pop into your mind without warning and may seem like normal thoughts, because they're so familiar to you. Because of this, you'll need to exercise some thought vigilance—which means staying aware of your thoughts and pulling the alarm when one of these myths presents itself.

TESTING THE VALIDITY OF YOUR THOUGHT MYTHS

Your next step will be to examine each myth, analyze its true worth, and come up with a healthy alternative by putting it to the "Challenging Your Thought Myths" test. The worksheet on the opposite page takes you through the process step by step.

For example, suppose that you gained a pound this week,

CHALLENGING YOUR THOUGHT MYTHS

The following worksheet will help you refute a Thought Myth that has been holding you back and contributing to your Runaway Eating cycle.

Identify one of your Thought Myths:

_____

Now challenge this Thought Myth by answering the following questions:

1. What evidence supports the thought?

_____

2. What alternative views are there (evidence against the thought)?

_____

_____

_____

3. What kinds of thoughts, feelings, and behaviors does the thought provoke?

_____

_____

_____

4. What kind of Thought Myth is this?

_____

5. Replace your Thought Myth with a more rational thought.

_____

_____

despite your efforts to get your eating under control. In your frustration, you tell yourself, "I might as well give up and binge—I'll always be overweight." It's time to challenge that Thought Myth. Of course, it's true that you gained a pound—the scales don't lie. But then you start to explore alternative views. You recall that the high-salt meal you had last night may have left you bloated, and you remind yourself that bingeing will make everything worse. You realize that it is the Thought Myth that is causing your feelings of anger, self-pity, and depression, and you recognize the myth as all-or-nothing thinking. Finally, you replace the Thought Myth with a more rational thought, "I gained a pound this week, but that doesn't justify a binge. If I focus on healthy eating and moderate exercise, my appetite and body weight will stabilize at a healthy level, and I can get off this roller coaster."

Try the "Challenging Your Thought Myths" test with every one of your Thought Myths and find a new, healthy replacement thought for each. Then, the next time one of these myths pops into your mind, consciously replace it with the new thought. These new thoughts may feel alien to you, especially because the Thought Myths are so familiar and comfortable, but the more you practice, the easier it gets. Soon, your healthy thoughts will become as automatic as your old, unhealthy ones used to be.

REROUTING YOUR THOUGHTS

Another cognitive-behavioral technique that you might find helpful is the restructuring of your thoughts from their inception, a technique we call rerouting your thoughts. By breaking down all the elements that lead to an episode of Runaway Eating and putting them into chart form, you'll be able to see how your thoughts affect your behavior.

The "Before" Setup

To chart an episode of Runaway Eating, you need to begin with the cue that set it off. Take a look at the "Rerouting Your Thoughts—Sample Before" worksheet on page 132. Notice how the cue ("fight with my husband") prompted a Thought Myth ("I can't handle these feelings; eating something will make me feel better"), which prompted both physical responses (heart pounding, hands shaking, feeling hot and sweaty) and feelings (anger, feeling unappreciated, depression, tension). The resultant behavior (eating chips and three Fudgsicles) had both positive consequences (less angry, numb, stopped the fight) and negative consequences (ate loads of calories, felt depressed and sick, fight unresolved).

Now try charting one of your own Runaway Eating episodes. From the list of your Runaway Eating cues that you made in chapter 6 (see page 116), select one and think back to the thoughts, feelings, and behaviors that it set off. Then make two copies of the blank worksheet on page 136 and fill in one copy as follows. (You'll use the second copy in a moment.)

- ◆ Cue: What cue set off your unhealthy eating behaviors?
- ◆ Thought Myth: What Thought Myths came to mind as a direct result of the cue?
- ◆ Physical responses: How did your body react to the cue or the Thought Myth? (Reactions might include tense muscles, butterflies in stomach, tears, or a pounding heart.)
- ◆ Feelings: What emotions came up in response to the cue or the Thought Myth?
- ◆ Behavior: What did you do in response to the thoughts, physical responses, or feelings?
- ◆ Consequences: What were the positive results of this behavior? What were the negative results?

REROUTING YOUR THOUGHTS—SAMPLE "BEFORE"

CUE	THOUGHT MYTHS	BEHAVIOR	CONSEQUENCES
Fight with my husband about my spending habits.	**THOUGHT MYTHS** I can't handle these feelings. Eating something will make me feel better. **PHYSICAL RESPONSES** Heart pounding; hands shaking; feeling hot and sweaty. **FEELINGS** Angry; feeling unappreciated; sad; tense.	Ate entire bag of potato chips plus 3 Fudgsicle bars.	**Positive** Was less angry; felt sort of numb; kept me from continuing the fight. **Negative** Ate loads of calories, and now I'll probably gain weight; felt really depressed, sick, and sick of myself; fight still unresolved.

The "Rerouted" Setup

Read through the "Rerouting Your Thoughts—Sample After" worksheet on page 134 and note how a simple change in thinking led to a much more healthy outcome. The cue ("fight with my husband") was the same, but it prompted a healthier thought ("I'm angry, but I'm going to sort through my feelings"), which in turn helped ease the physical responses (heart pounding and hands shaking) and led to some positive feelings (being calm and in control). The resultant behavior (writing a letter, then tearing it up; having a rational discussion) had positive consequences (increased insight into thoughts; better communication with husband) and only minor negative consequences (it's harder to sort out thoughts and feelings than it is to binge).

Now it's your turn to restructure the Thought Myth you recorded earlier. Get out your second copy of the blank worksheet and fill it in as follows:

- Cue: Put in the same cue as before.
- New healthy thought: Write down a rational, healthy alternate thought that could be substituted for the old Thought Myth. (See your "Challenging Your Thought Myths" worksheet on page 129.)
- Physical responses: How does your body respond to this new thought?
- Feelings: What emotions are associated with the new thought?
- Behavior: How might your behavior change in response to the new thought?
- Consequences: What would be the positive results of this behavior? What would be the negative results?

REROUTING YOUR THOUGHTS—SAMPLE "AFTER"

CUE

Fight with my husband about my spending habits.

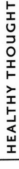

HEALTHY THOUGHT

I'm angry, but I'm not going to drown my feelings in food. I need to sort through my feelings. Then I'll have a better idea of what to do.

PHYSICAL RESPONSES

Heart pounding; hands shaking—at first; then a feeling of calm and control came over me.

FEELINGS

Calm; determined.

BEHAVIOR

Sat down and wrote a letter to my husband telling him just how I felt about his criticism of me, why I spend as much as I do, and where I thought we could cut back; tore up the letter; but had a calm, rational discussion about finances later. We came up with a cost-cutting plan that we think might work.

CONSEQUENCES

Positive

Was able to figure out how I felt and what I thought and communicate it; didn't rely on food to get me through a nonfood-related problem.

Negative

It's harder to do it this way than to just stuff my feelings down with food, but it's worth it.

How to Use the "Rerouting Your Thoughts" Worksheet

You can use the worksheet on page 136 in three ways.

Afterward. After you've experienced your next bout of Runaway Eating, fill out a worksheet and try to figure out what went wrong. How did your thoughts get you into trouble? At what point could you have changed directions?

During. The best time to figure out what's bringing on your Runaway Eating is right in the middle of an episode, when you can really tune in to what you're thinking and feeling. The next time you find yourself bingeing, purging, or restricting, stop for a minute and write down exactly what's going on, inside and outside. The insights you gain can be invaluable.

Before. Once you have some idea of what triggers your Runaway Eating, fill out the worksheet twice based on a typical cue or Thought Myth. The first time, jot down the way you usually react. The second time, write down a better way of handling the situation. By anticipating problem situations and arming yourself with a set of healthy thoughts that can replace old unhealthy ones, you'll be better prepared to deal with whatever comes up.

A DAY IN THE LIFE

Sometimes it's easier to figure out what's causing someone else's problems than it is to understand what's behind your own. Read through "Sheri's Story" on page 137 to try to identify the cues, thoughts, and feelings that fuel her Runaway Eating behaviors. Our analysis follows the story. Once you see what's driving Sheri's eating problems, you may be better able to figure out the forces behind your own.

REROUTING YOUR THOUGHTS WORKSHEET

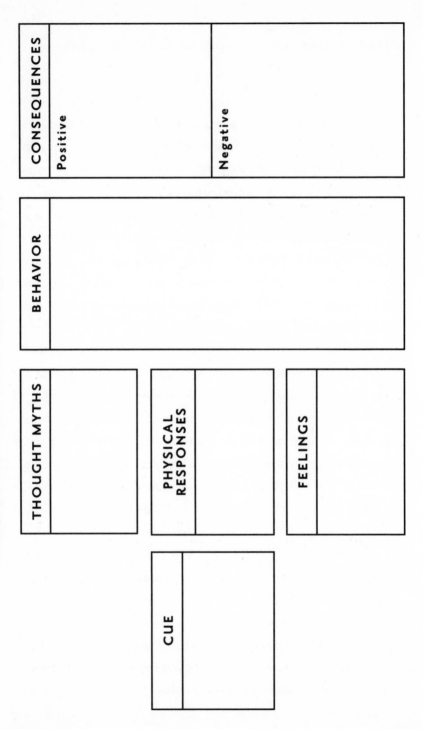

CUE

THOUGHT MYTHS

PHYSICAL RESPONSES

FEELINGS

BEHAVIOR

CONSEQUENCES

Positive

Negative

Sheri's Story

"I was 34 years old when I met my husband. I'd been working as a PR agent at a big New York fashion house for 8 years, but I quit once we were married because John made very good money as a set designer and he really didn't want me to work full-time. But because John was out on the road, I ended up spending an awful lot of time by myself with nothing much to do.

"My years in the fashion industry had taught me how important it is to be thin and to look hip. But after I quit working, some days I didn't even get dressed, and all that sitting around just made me want to eat. I had days when I watched DVDs from the time I got up until the time I went to bed, while I ate bags and bags of chips washed down with soda. It was depressing, but I couldn't muster the energy to do anything. I'd usually feel bad about indulging myself, though, and fast for a day or two.

"Finally, in order to get out of the house, I started making lunch dates with my old friends from work. I'd usually go without breakfast, drink a couple of martinis at the restaurant to loosen up, and eat a big restaurant lunch. Then I'd tell myself everything would be fine as long as I skipped dinner. But around 10:00 at night, I'd get hungry and eat whatever I could find—usually a couple of big bowls of ice cream with chocolate sauce, for starters.

"I gained 20 pounds during my first year of marriage, which made me feel unattractive. John got a permanent job in the city, so he was suddenly at home every night. He didn't say anything about my weight, but we sure weren't having much sex for newlyweds.

"Once he was no longer on the road, we developed a new routine: We started going out for dinner almost every night. I love good food, wine, and multicourse dinners. But at the same time, I knew I was getting as big as a house and couldn't afford to eat

THE ROLE OF THE MENTAL HEALTH PROFESSIONAL

Many people find that following our 8-point Runaway Eating plan is enough to help them regain control over their unhealthy eating habits. But others may find that they also need some form of face-to-face talk therapy with a mental health professional who can provide guidance and feedback.

A mental health professional can:

- Help you understand the origins of your Runaway Eating.
- Help treat coexisting conditions, such as depression, drug abuse, or anxiety disorders.
- Help you identify the cues, thoughts, and feelings that are contributing to your Runaway Eating behaviors.
- Show you how to replace unhealthy behaviors with healthy ones.
- Help make new ways of thinking a permanent part of your "thought library."

If you decide that working with a mental health professional would be beneficial to you, your next step should be to determine which type of professional can best serve your needs. Although anyone can call himself or herself a therapist and set up a practice, a licensed mental health professional who has

---

like that or I'd end up divorced. So I came up with a plan: I'd fast all day, then eat whatever I wanted at dinner—appetizer, soup or salad, entrée, and dessert, plus several glasses of wine.

"Unfortunately, even though I didn't eat anything but dinner, I was still gaining weight. It seemed like every time I stepped on the scale, the number was higher. This threw me into a panic. So I tried throwing up when I'd get home from the restaurant, but I couldn't make it work. That's when I decided on laxatives. Yeah, they gave me terrible diarrhea, and I had to keep increasing the dose, but I thought that if I sped the food through my body quickly enough,

been trained in the field of eating disorders may offer the best quality of care. Psychiatrists are medical doctors and, as such, are the only mental health professionals who can prescribe medication. Psychologists have earned either a master's degree or a doctoral degree in psychology, and social workers hold a master's or doctoral degree in social work.

Your choice of therapist should depend on both your needs and the therapist's qualifications. To find a qualified mental health professional, ask your doctor for a referral, or if there is a specialized eating disorders service near you, call for an evaluation or a referral. Be sure that the therapist is licensed to practice in your state, has a graduate degree from a reputable university, and has had experience in treating eating disorders. Once you get some names, make sure you take the time to interview all of them before you decide which (if any) is right for you.

Note: Seek help from a physician or mental health professional *immediately* if you are having suicidal thoughts, if you feel your depression or anxiety isn't improving, or if you have health problems related to your Runaway Eating.

I wouldn't get fat. Now I have to take 50 to 60 laxative pills a day to make my intestines work at all. And I'm not any skinnier."

———— ✿ ————

Sheri's thoughts and feelings trigger Runaway Eating at practically every turn. All of her "bandages" involve food (or alcohol) fixes that just increase the magnitude of her Runaway Eating problem.

Cued by boredom and isolation, Sheri becomes depressed and consoles herself with bags of chips and lots of soda while zoning out in front of the TV. Then she panics and feels guilty about the calorie overload, feelings that are fueled by thoughts like "It's important to be thin and look hip." These thoughts then lead to unhealthy behaviors like skipping breakfast when she plans to go out to lunch, forgoing dinner on the days when she thinks she's eaten too much, or fasting for days at a time. Restaurant food, alcohol, and the tension she feels when seeing old friends are additional cues, triggering negative thoughts about herself and her life, which she tries to numb with bingeing.

Unfortunately, the meal skipping and fasting just increase Sheri's depression and feelings of deprivation. Her hunger at the end of the day is the body cue that leads her to believe that it's okay to eat whatever she wants, so she starts in on the ice cream.

Sheri's weight gain of 20 pounds during her first year of marriage contributes to a worsening of her self-esteem; she feels unattractive. Her anxiety about her increased weight is worsened by thoughts like "I'm getting as big as a house" and "I can't afford to eat like this or I'll end up divorced." Her new habit of eating big restaurant dinners every night just exacerbates the problem. In an attempt to regain control of her eating, her weight, and her life, Sheri embarks on a brand-new pattern of bingeing and fasting.

But when she steps on the scale and sees that her weight has gone up instead of down, Sheri is catapulted into even more desperate weight-control methods—attempted vomiting and laxative abuse. Of course, neither prove to be the solution to her problems, because food, weight loss, diets, and overeating simply mask the much more complex problems that have yet to be addressed.

If there were any parts of Sheri's story that you identified with, use the strategies you learned in this chapter to come up with new, healthier alternatives to the Runaway Eating cycle. You *can* break the chain—and it starts when you take the first step.

CHAPTER 8

Transform Your Moods

You've seen how changing your thoughts can derail Runaway Eating. A change in thoughts translates to a change in feelings, which translates to a change in behavior. But can you change your feelings directly? Trying to force a good feeling on top of a bad one rarely works, because you really can't just command yourself to feel a certain way. Sometimes you may be able to bully yourself into behaving in a way that is inconsistent with your feelings (like touching a snake even though you are phobic), but that doesn't mean you aren't still scared to death!

Moods, however, are a different story. Although a feeling can be a single impulse or event ("I'm afraid of that spider"), a mood is an overall state of mind that results from a combination of thoughts, feelings, and the events around you ("I'm down in the dumps today"). Moods are great motivating forces in our lives. A confident mood will prompt us to strike out and do something different; a cautious mood will make us hunker down and beware. Angry moods make us want to fight or flee; affectionate moods incline us to draw closer. A score of moods can prompt Runaway Eating, including sadness, lethargy, loneliness, boredom, anxiety, frustration, and anger, to name just a few. Though feelings are hard to alter, you can do much to manage your moods, thereby short-circuiting the Runaway Eating cycle. It's not nearly as impossible or unnatural as it sounds; you already do it all the time—usually without even thinking about it.

THE BAD MOOD: A LOW-ENERGY, HIGH-TENSION KIND OF THING

Robert E. Thayer, Ph.D., author of *The Origin of Everyday Moods*, points out that most bad moods result from a combination of low energy and high tension levels. When your energy flags and tension gets the upper hand, you'll find yourself experiencing physical symptoms like fatigue, knotted muscles, tooth grinding, headaches, hyperventilation, or a down feeling.

This "energy down/tension up" imbalance is easy to see in the case of sadness. Let's say you've just lost your job and it's your first weekday morning at home with nothing to do. Your energy level is at a low ebb, maybe so low that you can't even get out of bed. At the same time, your tension levels (the anger, frustration, or fear within) are probably quite high, sapping your energy even further. This combination of low energy and high tension leaves you with a true face-pressed-into-the-mattress sadness. If you could somehow boost your energy and lessen your tension, your low mood would probably vanish, or at least recede.

But what about other bad moods? Aren't some of them, like anger, supercharged with energy? You might feel as though you have boundless energy when you're angry, but what you're really experiencing is boundless tension. Have you ever noticed how little you can actually achieve when you're ready to blow your stack? That's because your physiological responses (skyrocketing heart rate, blood pressure, blood sugar, and muscle tension, to name a few) take a great deal of energy to maintain, leaving you with a limited supply of constructive energy. Thus, you find yourself too keyed up to do much but pace back and forth through the living room. If you could just bring those tension levels back down to normal, your energy levels would automatically rise, and you'd be able to concentrate on the task at hand. Getting rid of a bad mood, then, is a two-step process: You must raise your energy levels and reduce your tension, nervousness, and anxiety.

MOOD REGULATION

When your energy is low and your tension is high, you may suddenly get the urge to drink a cup of coffee, take deep breaths, have a glass of wine, listen to music, see a movie, smoke a cigarette, or eat a hot fudge sundae. Although you may not know why you're doing these things (you just "feel like it"), your mind and body are trying to pump up your energy and release tension in a nearly unconscious process called mood regulation.

Mood-regulating behaviors are important, for they can keep us on an even keel, physically, mentally, and emotionally. Thanks to these behaviors, we don't stay sad or angry forever; we eventually get over whatever was bothering us. Often mood-regulating behaviors have an immediate effect: The good feelings increase, and the bad feelings dissipate. We like these results, so we repeat the behaviors. And over time, with enough repetition and reinforcement, the behaviors become habits.

Some of our mood-regulating habits are positive and health promoting. Activities such as exercising, using relaxation techniques, and meditating, for example, not only transform bad moods into good ones but also confer other physical, mental, and emotional benefits. Other mood-regulating behaviors may have less positive effects but cause no real harm if used in moderation, such as pampering yourself, watching television, or drinking a caffeinated beverage. But these behaviors can become harmful if they are overused (think of the shopaholic who can't stop buying things) or have unhealthy side effects (as seen in alcohol abuse).

Food as a Mood Regulator

Just about all of us use food to regulate our moods, at least to a certain extent. We drink coffee to get rolling in the morning, or we raid the pantry when we're bored. We eat chocolate when we're sad and drink hot milk when we want to wind down. But Runaway Eaters tend to rely much more heavily on food or food-related behaviors to regulate their moods. Eating a half gallon of ice cream can become a response to feeling blue; purging, a response to agitation or anger; scarfing down two bags of potato chips with dip, a response to boredom or emptiness; going on the latest fad diet, a response to anxiety. For the Runaway Eater, food or food-related behaviors have become her standard way of handling uncomfortable moods. She heads for a Starbucks when she's tired; she eats a box of doughnuts when she's upset about her boss; she goes on a strict diet when she's worried about aging. But whether it's coffee, doughnuts, or dieting, the motivation behind these behaviors is the same—all are desperate attempts to get rid of bad moods.

What's behind Your Eating?

When you're in the middle of a Runaway Eating episode, more likely than not you're using food or food-related activities to try to get rid of a bad mood—to boost your energy levels, ease your tension levels, or both. For example, if your mother-in-law calls to say she's coming to stay for a week and you eat four candy bars immediately after you hang up the phone, it's pretty clear that you're trying to relieve high levels of tension. On the other hand, if you wake from a nap and go straight to the kitchen in search of something sweet, your body is telling you that you need to increase your energy. And finally, if you're not getting enough sleep and you can't seem to stop eating, it's likely that you're trying to use food to boost your sagging energy levels and relieve the tension that's keeping you up at night.

When bad moods arise, your body realizes that your energy and tension levels are off-kilter, so it sends a message to your brain that something needs to be done. Food and food-related behaviors can temporarily increase energy and release tension, at least to some extent, thereby helping you to regain emotional balance. That's why when you're tired, sad, frustrated, or angry, you automatically head for something sweet and starchy. Sugar boosts your energy, and foods with a high carbohydrate content can influence levels of serotonin, a neurotransmitter that affects both mood and appetite. When you're headed for the cookie jar, you probably don't know why Oreos improve your mood—you just know they work and you crave them. You're trying to get rid of your bad mood and replace it with a good one by eating cookies. But herein lies an important distinction: *It's not the Oreos that you're after. It's the energy boost and the tension release.*

Following this logic, if there were some other way you could increase your energy or relieve your tension, you could exchange bad moods for good ones without the calorie load and guilty feelings that come with an Oreo binge. The good news is you can. Many, many behaviors can raise your energy, ease your tension, and turn bad moods into good ones, often even more effectively than food. As it turns out, food doesn't really work very well as a mood regulator. The results can be minimal and are usually fleeting, and the side effects are often most unpleasant. But which behaviors work better?

CHANGING A BAD MOOD INTO A GOOD ONE

The list of mood-regulating strategies people use is long and varied, and includes the following:

- Avoiding the cause of the bad mood
- Calling, seeing, or talking to a friend
- Doing anything that's fun or pleasant
- Doing chores
- Drinking alcohol
- Drinking coffee or another caffeinated beverage
- Eating
- Engaging in a hobby
- Engaging in religious or spiritual activities
- Exercising
- Having sex
- Keeping busy
- Listening to music
- Looking for the humor in the situation
- Meditating
- Pampering yourself
- Practicing relaxation techniques, such as yoga, meditation, or deep breathing
- Practicing stress-management techniques, such as biofeedback, positive thinking, or self-massage
- Putting it all in perspective
- Reading or writing

- Relaxing in a hot tub
- Resting or sleeping
- Screaming, crying, or otherwise venting
- Seeing a movie or watching TV
- Shopping
- Smoking cigarettes
- Spending time alone
- Taking a bath or shower, or splashing your face with water
- Taking a drive, a walk, or otherwise changing location
- Thinking about something else
- Thinking positively
- Trying to figure out what's causing the mood
- Using drugs
- Visiting a friend

Some of these mood-altering strategies are behaviors, like taking a drive or drinking alcohol, and some are thinking strategies, like trying to figure out what's causing the problem. To learn which strategies were most effective, Dr. Robert Thayer asked 308 people between the ages of 16 and 89 what they did when bad moods struck. Then he and his team analyzed the answers to see which strategies were best: that is, which were felt to be the most effective, which were best for raising energy, and which were best for reducing tension. The winning strategies (the ones they thought were good mood regulators, energy producers, and tension relievers) were exercising and listening to music. The runners-up were calling, seeing, or talking to someone, and doing chores. It's interesting to note that while eating made it onto the list of most effective strategies for raising energy, it had a fairly low rating when it came to altering mood.

A MOOD-ALTERING SUBSTANCE: MUSIC!

Although many kinds of music can offer therapeutic benefits, the kind that evokes pleasant memories from the past can be especially good at erasing a bad mood. Put on one of these oldies-but-goodies, and see if you don't feel better right away.

To increase energy and pump up your mood:
"Ain't Too Proud to Beg"—The Temptations
"Born to Be Wild"—Steppenwolf
"Dancing in the Street"—Martha Reeves and the Vandellas
"Gimme Some Lovin' "—The Spencer Davis Group
"Good Lovin' "—The Young Rascals
"Magic Carpet Ride"—Steppenwolf
"Ride My Seesaw"—The Moody Blues
"Surfin' USA"—The Beach Boys
"Time Has Come Today"—The Chambers Brothers

To get inspired:
"A Beautiful Morning"—The Rascals
"Classical Gas"—Mason Williams
"Feelin' Stronger Every Day"—Chicago
"Getting Better"—The Beatles
"Peace Train"—Cat Stevens
Theme from movie *2001: A Space Odyssey*
"Up, Up and Away"—The Fifth Dimension
"What's Going On?"—Marvin Gaye

The Most Effective Mood Regulators

Let's take a closer look at the top ways to turn a bad mood into a good one, to discover what makes them so effective.

Exercise is one of the simplest and best ways to reduce stress, tension, anxiety, and fatigue. When you're under stress (and who

To relax or calm hyperactivity:
"Crystal Blue Persuasion"—Tommy James and the Shondells
"For Emily, Whenever I May Find Her"—Simon and Garfunkel
"Groovin' "—The Young Rascals
"Into the Mystic"—Van Morrison
"Just My Imagination (Running Away with Me)"—The Temptations
"Nights in White Satin"—The Moody Blues

To ease sadness or boredom:
"Bridge over Troubled Water"—Simon and Garfunkel
"Brown-Eyed Girl"—Van Morrison
"Get Ready"—The Temptations
"All Shook Up"—Elvis Presley
"It's Your Thing"—The Isley Brothers
"Rock around the Clock"—Bill Haley and His Comets
"When I'm 64"—The Beatles

Of course, oldies aren't the only kind of music that can ease tension, energize you, or turn a bad mood around. Look through your CD collection or take a trip to your local music store and assemble a list of your own favorites. Make categories of songs you can play for every mood. Keep them at hand and pop in a tape or CD next time you're feeling out of sorts. Even better, try exercising to music. Dancing, doing jazzercise, walking with headphones on, or just working out while listening to music that gets you going can all be great mood elevators.

isn't?), your body releases high-voltage chemicals that send it into high gear. Exercise offers a natural outlet for these chemicals, releasing tension in the skeletal muscles, discharging pent-up frustration, and bringing your body back to its normal state. It also boosts energy by increasing blood circulation; releasing endorphins; improving elimination through the skin, lungs, and bowels;

reducing insomnia; improving blood sugar regulation; and enhancing oxygenation of the blood and brain, which increases alertness and concentration. Those who exercise regularly also enjoy less depression, a greater control over feelings of anxiety, improved self-esteem, and a lessened dependency on alcohol and drugs. (For more on exercise, see chapter 9.)

Listening to music can help energize the physical body, calm anger, release tension, lessen boredom, relieve depression, decrease fear, and lessen grief. It can also inspire feelings of strength, courage, love, and devotion; stimulate clear thinking; and assist in meditation and relaxation. Dr. Thayer suggests that familiar music may call up a conditioned response because it's linked to pleasant memories, and that rhythmic music relieves tension by getting you to move your body. But no matter why or how it works, music can do plenty to dispel a bad mood and make you feel better.

It's interesting to note that calling, seeing, or talking to someone and doing chores also rated high on the mood-regulation scale, second only to exercise and listening to music. It certainly makes sense to try to connect with others when you feel down. Talking over your problems with a good friend gets your mind off your troubles: It's soothing, reassuring, and distracting, and it's also an excellent way to reduce nervousness, tension, and anxiety. People who have recovered from serious problems like drug addiction or eating disorders often say that the single most important factor in their recovery was having someone who believed in them, loved them, and didn't give up on them. As Mother Teresa once said, "The most important medicine is tender love and care."

As for doing chores to make yourself feel better, just getting up off the couch and moving around can get your blood moving, work off some tension, and start to raise your energy levels. Like socializing, doing chores can be distracting: It can short-circuit tension-producing thoughts and give you a different focus. Most chores involve rhythmic, repetitive actions (scrubbing, vacuuming, folding laundry, and so on) that can help calm the mind, control anxiety-producing thoughts, and ease tension. However, for those who drive themselves to complete chore after chore, or insist on doing each one perfectly, doing chores can greatly increase tension and make a bad mood worse. If this sounds like you, doing chores would obviously not be a good choice as a mood regulator in your case.

GIVING A BAD MOOD THE BOOT

Before you can change your moods, you must first become aware of them. Your "Daily Logs for Self-Monitoring" and "Rerouting Your Thoughts" worksheets from chapters 6 and 7 will come in handy for this. Take another look at them, paying particular attention to the feelings that preceded incidents of Runaway Eating. What moods were you trying to regulate? Loneliness, fatigue, anxiety, tension, sadness, boredom? How well did your Runaway Eating behaviors regulate these moods? Chances are they weren't very effective at all. They may have worked sometimes but only temporarily. And most likely, they led to other moods that were just as destructive and painful as the original ones. The next time you get the urge to engage in Runaway Eating, ask yourself, "What mood am I trying to change?"

Now that you know which mood-regulating strategies work best, you're in a good position to pick some Mood Transformers—behaviors that you can use instead of Runaway Eating to change bad moods into better ones. Think about the various ways you try to change your mood—and then think about the strategies you *could* use to change your mood. Which ones attack the problem of low energy and high tension levels most directly? Exercising, positive thinking, looking for the humor in the situation, and doing chores are often helpful in rebalancing energy and tension levels. Distracting yourself by listening to music, engaging in a hobby, and taking a walk are also helpful. Much less effective are venting, looking for instant gratification, distracting yourself with a television show or a movie, and just simply avoiding the situation.

Remember, the key to getting rid of a bad mood is figuring out what will crank up your energy level while letting go of tension. Brainstorm which strategies do this best for you and then write them below.

Mood Transformers: Ways to Get Rid of a Bad Mood

Activities that increase energy and decrease tension:

_____   _____

_____   _____

_____   _____

_____   _____

_____   _____

Ways to increase my energy:

_____   _____

_____   _____

_____   _____

_____   _____

_____   _____

Ways to relieve my tension:

_____   _____

_____   _____

_____   _____

_____   _____

_____   _____

Once you have created your Mood Transformers list, try out these behaviors one at a time when you're not having the urge to engage in Runaway Eating, so that you can get accustomed to them. That way, when you do have Runaway Eating urges later on, you'll be able to turn to these behaviors, and they'll feel like old friends.

COMBATING THE NEXT RUNAWAY EATING URGE

Up until now, Runaway Eating has been your default, your automatic reaction to unpleasant emotions. Reprogramming yourself is going to take time, effort, and awareness. So it's a given that when the old food-related urges arise, you'll automatically want to react in the old ways. To break the Runaway Eating habit, you'll need to do your best to resist those urges and substitute new thoughts and new behaviors—especially those from your Mood Transformers list—for the old ones. You may not always succeed, but the more often you try, the easier the process will become. Let's take a look at some additional strategies that can help you through this process, allowing you to eventually trade in your old destructive habits for healthy new ones.

Fighting the Urge

When a Runaway Eating urge arises, do the following three things.

Wait a minute. When an urge arises, it's natural to want to satisfy it immediately. By consciously pausing for 1 minute before you do anything, you can short-circuit the "automatic" part of Runaway Eating and exert a certain amount of control over your actions. This also gives you time to think about what's really going on and to put some of your tools to work. Focus on your thoughts and feelings. Think about the consequences of your Runaway Eating behaviors. Then try thought restructuring, using relaxation techniques, or substituting an alternative behavior.

Ask yourself what mood you are trying to change. It's not the food you want, it's the change of mood. Try to determine what's really going on—then find another way to transform that mood.

Ride the wave. Urges have peaks and troughs, just like waves. Although you may think your urge will get stronger the longer you wait, it actually gets weaker. But you won't know this until you try. Do something else while you ride it out.

Refocusing Your Energy

Many Runaway Eaters spend a tremendous amount of time and energy engaging in unhealthy eating behaviors. It's not only the time that's spent bingeing, purging, or exercising excessively but also the time spent obsessing about food, diets, and body shape or size; planning meals; cooking; poring over the latest diet book; and so on. For some people, thoughts of food, eating, and dieting literally dominate their day. But when eating behaviors stop being a major focus, the Runaway Eater will need to put all that energy into some other activities.

To avoid falling back into old habit patterns, make a list of 10 things that you can do instead of engaging in Runaway Eating. Look at your Mood Transformers list to remind yourself of your best ways of raising energy and lowering tension. Then select 10 that you think you can substitute for Runaway Eating behaviors. But this time, make them very specific. For example, instead of writing down "Listen to music," write "Put on a Diana Krall CD." Instead of "Do chores," write "Vacuum the living room." Instead of "Call a friend," write "Call Bob." Being specific is important because when the old urges strike, it can be hard to think clearly or act rationally, despite your best intentions. You want to present yourself with a very clear, concise message so that you don't have to think. It will all be there in front of you.

You may want to have separate lists for different places. For example, if you tend to do your Runaway Eating at work, you want alternative behaviors that you can do at your desk, such as "Take 10 deep breaths," "Get up and stretch," or "Call my best friend." If you're an at-home Runaway Eater, your list may include such things as "Do my nails," "Wash my hair," or "Listen to a progressive relaxation tape."

Here are a few more examples for inspiration.

At-work alternative behaviors:

- Call a friend
- Read a magazine
- Do isometric exercises in your chair
- Take 10 deep breaths (in through your nose and out through your mouth)
- Take a walk
- Chat with a coworker

- Drink a glass of water
- Get up and stretch
- Play computer games
- Surf the Internet

At-home alternative behaviors:

- Play with your kids
- Take a shower
- Do a craft
- Walk the dog
- Rearrange the furniture
- Exercise to music
- Take a nap
- Put on your favorite CD
- Meditate
- Have friends over
- Read a book
- Do some gardening

Once you've made your very specific list of alternative behaviors, copy each one onto a 3- by 5-inch index card. We call these U-Turn cards, because their simple suggestions may be just the little bit of impetus you need to get off the Runaway Highway. You can keep them in your purse, in your kitchen, on your desk at work, or in any other place where you're at high risk for Runaway Eating. A U-Turn card is a simple tool that can help you transform your mood, refocus your purpose, and break your old destructive habit patterns. Whenever you feel your old Runaway Eating habits taking hold, grab your cards. Sometimes, just a slight refocusing of your energy and your thought patterns will be enough to get you back on track.

Validations

Most of us are great at criticizing ourselves and sending a steady stream of negative self-statements through our heads. That's why it's vitally important to focus on your many positive qualities—to validate yourself—in order to have the ammunition to fight off these negative thoughts and feelings.

You can start by making a list of positive things about yourself that focus on your inner qualities. Are you a good listener? Are you generous? Are you creative? Are you a good friend? Think of at least 10 of your best qualities, then write each one on the list below, preceded by the words "I am."

1. I am _____.

2. I am _____.

3. I am _____.

4. I am _____.

5. I am _____.

6. I am _____.

7. I am _____.

8. I am _____.

9. I am _____.

10. I am _____.

Now, choose one validation per week and work with it. Look for examples in your life that support it, and repeat the validation to yourself when you do something that confirms it. For example, tell yourself, "I really am a good listener," when you've taken the time to listen to a friend or family member confide a problem. This approach can help you recognize and reinforce some of your own distinctive qualities. You truly are a unique individual with very special attributes—you just need to hear it more often! Add new validations to your list over time, and review the entire list at least once a day.

Affirmations

While validations recognize your inner qualities, affirmations are strong, positive self-statements that you don't believe are true but you wish were true. However, the more you repeat them to yourself, the truer they become. For example, you might say to yourself, "I have control over food." Or "I like myself no matter what I weigh." Or "I eat only when I'm hungry." Affirmations are replacement thoughts for the negative self-statements and Thought Myths that can run through your head like a ticker tape when you're caught up in Runaway Eating. Make a list of 10 affirmations by using the examples below or (even better) making up your own.

Examples:

- I accept myself no matter how much I weigh.
- I have a high opinion of myself.
- I may not always like what I do, but I always like who I am.
- I am happy.
- I have control over food.
- My opinion of myself doesn't depend on what others think of me.
- I treat my body with respect and love.
- I can completely change my old destructive habits.

- I am a lovable and special person.
- I can eat what I want and still love myself.
- I am proud of who I am.
- I am good to myself.
- I am in control of my life.
- I can make it through any situation.
- I can regain control even if I've engaged in out-of-control behaviors.
- I can achieve whatever I set out to do.

1. _____.

2. _____.

3. _____.

4. _____.

5. _____.

6. _____.

7. _____.

8. _____.

9. _____.

10. _____.

As with the validations, focus on one affirmation per week, while thinking about what you can do to make the affirmation into a reality and what might be standing in your way. Read all your affirmations aloud at least once a day. The more you repeat them (either aloud or to yourself), the more they will become true for you.

CHAPTER 9

Alleviate Anxiety

While women have always had plenty to do during their midlife years, life has never been more stressful or more complicated than it is today. Ours is the first generation expected to take on both breadwinning and family responsibilities—a tall order. You're most likely raising children or teenagers, caring for ailing parents, working full-time, rising to challenges in your career, and running a household. To ratchet up your stress levels even further, you may be dealing with perimenopause or menopause, divorce, single motherhood, work overload (no doubt about this one!), frustrations at work, and qualms about aging in our youth-obsessed culture. If you often feel nervous, worried, fearful, tense, or uneasy—or it seems to you that your life is spiraling out of control—join the club!

Anxiety is apprehension, agitation, fear, or unease that arises when you feel there is some kind of danger or threat just around the corner. That threat could be something as specific as a job interview or as general as the day-to-day uncertainties of life. And just anticipating this threat can cause more anxiety than the threat itself. Whatever the cause, anxiety triggers certain physical, mental, and emotional symptoms, such as sweating, worrying, and exag-

SIGNS OF ANXIETY

Anxiety affects the way you think, the way you feel physically, and the way you behave. Any of the following can be signs of the anxiety response.

Anxious Thoughts

- You think you just can't cope.
- You worry about pleasing others.
- You're worried that you aren't in control (of your eating, your weight, or your life in general).
- You worry about having to go past the bakery section of the grocery store.
- You're afraid of losing your looks, vitality, and value as you age.
- You magnify the importance of the bad things that happen.
- You live in the future and predict the worst.
- You must be perfect; any mistake equals failure.
- You have a hard time concentrating; your thoughts race.
- You worry that you might get trapped or would be unable to escape from a place or situation.

Anxious Physical Feelings

- Your heart races.
- You feel shaky or dizzy.
- You have butterflies, or your stomach feels upset.
- You flush or blush.
- You perspire a lot.
- You feel a choking sensation or a tightening in your chest.
- Your muscles are tense.
- Your breathing is shallow and rapid.
- You are restless and may have a tremor.
- You have a panicky feeling.

Anxious Behaviors

- You avoid going to social events.
- You avoid feared events or objects, such as speaking in public or spiders.
- You unconsciously tap your fingers or your feet.
- You bite your fingernails or pick at your fingers.
- When you find yourself in a situation that makes you anxious, you leave.
- You find yourself eating more or less than usual.
- You don't take risks, even "reasonable" ones.
- You feel immobilized or unable to act.

gerated fear. When your anxious feelings occur frequently, last a long time, don't go away, or are so severe that they interfere with your ability to function, they may have progressed to an anxiety disorder.

THE LINK BETWEEN ANXIETY AND RUNAWAY EATING

Runaway Eating is triggered by a combination of physiological, psychological, and social factors, so we really can't place the blame for it on anxiety alone. Clinical studies show, however, that more than half of the women who have true anorexia nervosa have suffered from an anxiety disorder at some point during their lives. As for bulimia, in the majority of cases, anxiety disorders are present before the eating disorder emerges, causing researchers to suggest that anxiety disorders may be a risk factor for both anorexia and bulimia nervosa.

But it's not just anorexia nervosa and bulimia nervosa that are linked to anxiety. High levels of anxiety greatly increase the risk of developing eating problems at any level. This makes sense, as we've already seen that Runaway Eating is often fueled by a desire to regulate unpleasant emotions; in other words, Runaway Eaters diet, eat, exercise excessively, or purge to try to blunt bad moods. As we discussed in chapter 8, one of the defining features of a bad mood is a high level of tension, or anxiety, and the need to ease this tension is a prime motivating force behind Runaway Eating. So although anxiety by itself doesn't necessarily cause this behavior, it certainly plays an important role in bringing on and maintaining eating problems in most women.

Experts estimate that 80 to 90 percent of food binges are triggered by anxiety, tension, and other negative feelings. And we can clearly see this in the dieter whose tension levels skyrocket as she carefully monitors every bite of food and fights the urge to eat. Often the stress gets to be too much for her, so she lets go and binges just to relieve some tension. But we also see this in the woman who binges because she's keyed up from a stressful day, or in the woman who binges and then purges to get rid of the intense anxiety she feels about taking in too many calories. Anxiety also plagues those who binge without purging, as they worry about a binge-related weight gain.

In short, trying to follow a restrictive diet, bingeing, or getting caught in a binge/purge cycle can create a perpetual state of anxiety. You can find yourself afraid of food, your body, rejection by others, or generally just not being good enough.

Fortunately, there are numerous strategies you can use to release and reduce tension and lower your anxiety level, which will help you control your Runaway Eating. In the remainder of this chapter, we'll discuss the strategies we believe are the most helpful.

EXERCISE: THE NUMBER ONE ANXIETY BUSTER

The kind of exercise that is most effective for easing anxiety is aerobic exercise, which includes activities like brisk walking, jogging, running, tennis, basketball, skating, racquetball, continuous dancing, and cycling. Besides strengthening your heart, improving your lung capacity, and burning calories, aerobic (or cardio) exercise relieves muscle tension, burns up stress hormones, and stimulates the release of endorphins, the body's feel-good hormones. And by increasing oxygenation of the blood as well as blood flow to the brain, exercise increases your alertness and ability to concentrate.

Although exercise in moderate amounts can effectively relieve tension, too much can have the reverse effect. Excessive exercising—exercising beyond what is healthy, for more than an hour every day, for the sole purpose of weight loss—can become an obsessively driven behavior and can escalate both anxiety and tension. If you exercise more often and more intensely than necessary to maintain good health, if you beat yourself up emotionally when you miss a workout, if you continue to work out even when you're injured, or if your work, family life, or relationships are suffering because of the amount of time you devote to exercise, you're doing too much.

Elements of a Good Exercise Plan

Aerobic exercise is great, but it is most effective as part of a larger plan that includes five basic elements.

Warmup. Get your circulation going and increase the temperature in your muscles by doing 5 to 10 minutes of mild warmup exercises, such as moderate to brisk walking, easy jogging, jumping rope, or jumping jacks. This will get your body ready to move and help prevent injuries.

Aerobic exercise. Once you've broken a sweat, it's time to increase the intensity and speed up your heart and breathing rates with some jogging, running, continuous dancing, cycling, or whatever suits your fancy. To make sure you're working within the right range—that is, hard enough to get the benefits but not so hard that you risk injury—try the talk-sing test. Can you talk to a friend in short sentences without gasping for breath? If not, slow down a little. Are you able to sing while you're exercising? If you can, you're not working hard enough. Pace yourself so that you can talk but not sing.

We recommend doing some kind of aerobic exercise every other day for 20 to 30 minutes. If you're just beginning an exercise program, start with 5 to 10 minutes a day and gradually work your way up.

Strengthening exercises. These exercises increase the force that your muscles can exert (strength) and the length of time that they can do so (endurance). To strengthen your muscles, you must pit them against another force, whether it's gravity, weights, water, or your own body weight. Weight lifting, isometric exercises (such as putting your palms together and pushing), swimming, pushups, and leg lifts are different kinds of strengthening exercises. Do a 10- to 15-minute session of strengthening exercises every other day, gradually building up to 20 to 30 minutes. Alternate the days you do your aerobic workout with the days you do your strength-training workout.

Stretching. These exercises increase the elasticity of your muscles and the range of motion of your joints. Stretching is recommended after aerobic exercise and after weight lifting as well. Stretching is also a great way to relieve stress and muscle tension and increase relaxation. But to avoid injury, stretch slowly and carefully; it's a good idea to pick up a book on proper stretching techniques or consult a fitness trainer before you begin. (We recommend *Essential Stretch,* by Michelle LeMay. See Recommended Reading and Resources on page 271 for more information on the book.) A 10- to 15-minute stretching session done every other day can help alleviate your anxiety. If you find it helps you a lot, you might consider stretching every day.

Cooldown. This is the reverse of the warmup session, and you may even do the same exercises, if you like. But instead of speeding up your body, you want to slow it down. Include a 5-minute cooldown after every exercise session. The cooldown period is a great time to do a little more stretching, now that your muscles will be nice and warmed up.

Finally, keep in mind that it doesn't matter how great an exercise plan might be—if you don't enjoy it, you're not going to do it. The trick is to find something you really like and will do regularly. Taking a brisk walk around the neighborhood every evening will do a lot more to relieve your tension than a 10-mile run every other week. Dance, walk, run, ride a bike, or swim—if that's what makes you feel good—but do it often.

RELAXATION TECHNIQUES THAT SOOTHE AWAY TENSION

Deep breathing, yoga, meditation, tai chi, visualization, prayer, and other activities that help you slow down, center yourself, and calm both your body and your mind are excellent ways to relieve anxiety. Sensual pleasures, such as warm baths and aromatherapy, are also wonderful antidotes to stress and can lower your blood pressure, reduce tension, and almost instantly make you feel better.

Of all the many wonderful relaxation techniques, three deserve special mention because they are at the core of most stress-reduction programs: deep breathing, progressive muscle relaxation, and body scanning. (For information on other relaxation techniques, consult the books listed in Recommended Reading and Resources on page 271.)

Deep breathing. When you're anxious, angry, or in pain, you tend to take in air in quick, short, shallow breaths. You may even hold your breath for short periods of time. This kind of breathing actually increases anxiety, panic attacks, muscle tension, depression, headaches, and fatigue. Conversely, when you're relaxed and feeling good, each breath is much deeper, longer, and more regular, the kind of breathing that encourages relaxation, tension release, and quieting of the mind. Just by practicing deep breathing techniques, you can enhance your physical and psychological health and do much to control your anxiety.

First, find a quiet place where you can lie down or recline and won't be disturbed. Loosen any tight clothing and lie on your back on the floor (preferably on a mat), with your knees bent and the soles of your feet flat on the floor, about a foot apart. Place one palm lightly on your stomach just beneath your rib cage and the other palm on your chest.

Inhale deeply and slowly through your nose, allowing the air to go all the way down to your abdominal cavity. You should feel an expansion of your abdomen underneath your hand. Your chest, however, should expand very little. Once you've filled your abdominal cavity with air, fill your rib cage and then your chest. Hold your breath for a second or two, then slowly exhale through your mouth. Some people recommend saying the word "relax" in your head with every exhaled breath. That way, the sensation of exhaling through your mouth becomes paired with the thought of relaxing. Try to keep your body, face, jaw, and neck completely relaxed as you breathe. Repeat for a total of 10 breaths.

Once you get used to breathing into your abdomen, you can use this technique at any time during the day to relieve stress and tension, whether you're lying down, sitting, or even standing.

Progressive muscle relaxation. Many people go through the day unaware that they are carrying tension in certain muscles. This exercise puts you in touch with your muscles by systematically tensing and relaxing them.

Lie down on your back in a quiet place where you won't be disturbed, and take a few deep, relaxing breaths. As you let the rest of your body relax, inhale and tense the muscles in your right foot and lower leg. Hold for a couple of seconds, then exhale and release the tension completely, feeling the looseness in that foot and leg. Repeat with your other foot and leg. Slowly work your way up your body, tensing and releasing your thigh, hip and buttock, abdomen, and chest, isolating each muscle group as you go.

Move on to your lower arm, upper arm and shoulder, neck, and finally your face. Raise your eyebrows, frown, purse your lips, open your mouth wide. For the most relaxing effect, break this down into small muscle groups as well. Each time, notice the difference in your muscles when you tense them and then relax them completely. When you've tensed and released all the muscles in your body, take a few deep breaths and enjoy the feeling of being totally relaxed from head to toe.

Body scanning. With this exercise, you become more fully aware of each area of your body, focusing on any sensations that may exist and letting go of all tension.

Lie on your back and take a few deep breaths, which will automatically bring you into a more relaxed state. Then bring your attention to the bottoms of your feet. Mentally take inventory as to how they feel, noticing any sensations that might be present. Then breathe in slowly and imagine that your breath is flowing all the way down to the soles of your feet. Allow the soles of your feet to relax and "dissolve" as you exhale.

Next, bring your attention to the toes of your feet and repeat the process. Work all the way up your body, inhaling deeply, scanning for sensations. When you find tension, breathe into it and imagine the breath softening and loosening the tight, painful muscles. Then exhale and let the tension wash away.

The body-scanning process can take between 30 and 45 minutes and ideally should be done every day, especially when anxiety is a problem.

NATURAL SUPPLEMENTS FOR ANXIETY RELIEF

Natural supplements, such as vitamins, minerals, and herbs, may offer relief from anxiety symptoms and, in turn, help you to control your Runaway Eating. Here are a few to consider.

Multivitamin/mineral supplement. Chronic tension saps the body of vitamins and minerals, so you might want to take a multivitamin/mineral supplement that includes all the vitamins in the B complex (thiamin, riboflavin, niacin, B_6, B_{12}, folic acid, pantothenic acid, and biotin). Low levels of any of these can contribute to an anxious mood. Check to see if your multi contains the Daily Value of these vitamins; if it doesn't, consider purchasing one that does.

Antioxidants. Anxiety tends to weaken your immunity, but studies suggest that getting a good supply of the major antioxidants—8,400 micrograms of beta-carotene, 500 to 1,000 milligrams of vitamin C, 400 to 800 IU of vitamin E, and 100 to 200 micrograms of the mineral selenium—may help fortify your immune system, protect against cancer and heart disease, and ward off infections. Though all these antioxidants are available in supplement form, you can also increase your intake by eating antioxidant-rich foods. Good food sources of beta-carotene include cantaloupe, mangoes, carrots, butternut squash, spinach, and broccoli. Citrus fruits, strawberries, red peppers, kiwifruit, and papaya are excellent sources of vitamin C, and wheat germ oil, green leafy vegetables, nuts, and seeds are top sources of vitamin E. Good food sources of selenium include whole grains, poultry, meat, and fish.

Calcium and magnesium. A deficiency in calcium or magnesium can result in anxiety, fatigue, tension, or insomnia, so some doctors recommend taking calcium and magnesium supplements as a preventive strategy. Because most multivitamin/mineral supplements contain less than the daily requirement for calcium (1,000 milligrams) and magnesium (400 milligrams), additional supplements may be needed. But beware of taking too much of either mineral. Over time, taking more than 400 milligrams of supplementary magnesium per day can cause diarrhea, nausea, muscle weakness, and other problems. And regular ingestion of more than 2,000 milligrams of calcium per day can cause high levels of calcium in the urine, which could result in kidney stones.

It's best to get the calcium and magnesium you need every day by eating foods rich in these minerals, because they're better absorbed in food form. Then use supplements to make up the difference, if necessary. Top food sources of calcium include milk, yogurt, cheese, and canned salmon or sardines (with the bones). Top sources of magnesium are whole grain bread, peas, beans, and dark green leafy vegetables.

As for herbs, first a word of warning: A few herbs have been used successfully to treat anxiety, but they should be taken with caution. The wrong mixture of herbs, too much of any one kind of herb, or combining herbs with certain medications can be dangerous to your health. See your physician before beginning any regimen that includes herbs.

Although further research is needed to confirm their effectiveness and overall safety, the following three herbs have shown promise as anxiety relievers.

Chamomile *(Matricaria chamomilla)*. This herb has been used for centuries as a treatment for anxiety, tension, insomnia, back pain, and other ailments. There is no set dosage for chamomile, but some experts suggest drinking a cup of chamomile tea three times daily. Be careful, however, if you're allergic to ragweed, chrysanthemums, or other members of the aster or daisy families: Chamomile belongs to this family and can cause an allergic reaction. Start by taking the smallest possible dose, watching carefully for reactions.

Valerian *(Valerian officinalis)*. Valerian can exert a calming effect on the body, which is why the extract of the root of this plant is often recommended to ease anxiety, nervous tension, and the effects of stress. It's also a well-known sleep

(continued)

aid that may help decrease the time it takes to drift off, while improving overall sleep quality. Valerian is available in capsule form or as an extract, tincture, or tea. Don't take the herb if you are pregnant, are nursing, or have liver problems. Potential side effects include headaches, stomach upset, and (rarely) liver damage. High dosages of valerian can cause confusion, insomnia, hypersensitivity, hallucinations, or interactions with other drugs.

Kava *(Piper methysticum).* Kava is the most studied of the three anti-anxiety herbs. It's used in certain parts of the South Pacific as a ceremonial tranquilizing beverage, as well as a treatment for anxiety, insomnia, restlessness, and the effects of stress.

Several studies have shown that taking kava results in a significant decline in anxiety, and in some cases, this herb was found to be just as effective as standard anxiety medications. For example:

- In a 6-month study, 101 people with anxiety disorders were given either an extract of kava or a placebo. Those taking the kava extract showed a decrease in anxiety by the 8th week, a lessening that continued for the course of the study. Further, they didn't develop a tolerance to kava, a problem often seen with the use of traditional anxiety medications.

- Researchers pitted a proprietary brand of kava against a standard anxiety medication in a study of 38 patients with anxiety. The researchers concluded that kava was just as effective at easing anxiety as the drug.

Drowsiness, mild gastrointestinal problems, headaches, dizziness, equilibrium disturbances, and, in rare cases, allergic reactions involving the skin are all potential side effects of kava. People with liver disease or liver problems, or people who are taking drugs that affect the liver, should consult a physician before using kava-containing supplements. Using this herb in conjunction with alcohol, drugs that suppress the central nervous system, or other herbs with sedative properties increases the risk of side effects.

SIMPLIFY YOUR LIFE

One of the basic themes of this book is that we midlife women are so overloaded with responsibilities, jobs, and roles to fulfill that our anxiety levels skyrocket and we turn to food to find relief. That's why it's vitally important to pare down your responsibilities and find the most efficient and least stressful ways to accomplish your aims. To do this, you need to incorporate five strategies: prioritize, plan ahead, do one thing at a time, delegate, and learn to say no.

Prioritize. Make a list of the things in your life that really matter to you, then rank them in order of importance. Which comes first? Family? Good health? Wealth? Love? Friends? Now think about how much time you actually spend on each of these. Are you spending most of your time on the most important things in your life? If not, which activities, responsibilities, or duties can you scale down or even cross off your list?

Every day, draw up a list of things that must be done, and do the most important things first. If you consistently find that you can't get through your list, you're trying to do too much. Get help or get rid of some of your responsibilities—you can do only so much!

Plan ahead. When writing out your "to do" list, determine how much time you're willing to spend on each activity, and decide which ones you can skip—then cross them off. See if you can combine certain activities so that you can do them simultaneously, and look for shortcuts. Do your grocery shopping all at once, instead of making several quick trips a week. Lay out tomorrow's clothes, pack lunches, and get organized the night before to minimize chaos in the morning.

As difficult as it may seem in the midst of all that you do every day, try to schedule a little time to yourself. Some days this will be impossible—and the last thing you need is to feel guilty about it—but look for ways to give yourself a break. And when you do find some time to yourself, really savor it. If you find that you're continually shortchanged on "alone time," take it as a sign that you're doing too much.

Do one thing. We women often try to multitask, but we can end up frazzled, stressed out, and falling down on the job because it's impossible for anyone to focus well on several things at once. Try to zero in on one thing at a time as you go through your day. This will increase your efficiency and decrease your stress level. This is particularly important during the time you take for yourself. When you get a few moments of personal time, focus only on relaxing and centering yourself. Don't let your mind dwell on the grocery list, the children's homework, or what's for dinner. Multitasking becomes a liability when we need to let go and just relax.

Delegate. You may feel as if you're the only one who can handle certain tasks—and this may be true part of the time. But if you tend to feel this way about everything, you need to take a step back. Have a family meeting and divide the chores among all members. The laundry, cooking, dishes, cleaning, and gardening chores can all be shared—although you'll probably need to relax your standards a bit. You might also consider calling in reinforcements: Hiring a housecleaner, gardener, or maintenance person to help out occasionally can be well worth the cost.

Learn to say no. Those who suffer from anxiety often have trouble standing up for themselves, expressing their feelings, and saying no to the requests of others. They let others take advantage of them and disregard their needs and feelings. If this is your problem, make a conscious effort to be a little more direct and honest when expressing your thoughts and feelings. This doesn't mean that you should ignore the rights and feelings of others, but it's okay to clearly state what you can and can't do.

The next time someone asks you to do something you can't or don't want to do, try this: Look the person in the eye, explain that you understand why he's making such a request, and then either offer a brief explanation as to why you can't do it or just tell him that it's not possible. Either way, be clear about saying no. Although this person will probably try to persuade you to change your mind, remember: It's your right to refuse.

GET PLENTY OF HIGH-QUALITY SLEEP

One of the first places anxiety rears its ugly head is in the bedroom—and we're not talking about sex. When you're anxious, you may have trouble dropping off to sleep or staying asleep. Then you get anxious about not sleeping enough, which makes sleeping even more difficult. So even though getting plenty of sleep is critical to your mental health, it may be more elusive than ever when you're anxious and you really need it.

To improve your chances of getting a good night's sleep, follow these "good sleep" guidelines.

Figure out how much sleep you need. Experiment to determine how many hours you need (more than 8? fewer?) in order to feel refreshed, rested, and alert. Then organize your life so that you're getting that much.

Establish a sleeping schedule. Try to wake up and go to bed at the same time every day, even on weekends. Although you might enjoy sleeping in on the weekends, this throws off your internal clock.

Use your bed for sleep and sex only. Many of us watch TV, pay bills, eat, and write letters while in bed, which makes us associate the bed with activity. Reserve your bed solely for sleeping and sex, so you'll associate it with relaxation and sleep.

Get comfortable. If you wake up with a stiff neck or sore back, you may need a new mattress or pillow. Spend whatever it takes to get yourself the right pillow, mattress, or mattress cover. It's worth the money.

Relax before going to bed. Yoga, a warm bath, lovemaking, and relaxation exercises can help you decelerate and get ready for your descent into dreamland.

Stay cool, but don't get cold. Your body temperature needs to drop to a certain point before you can fall asleep. To help speed the process, try to keep your bedroom between 55° and 65°F, but keep a warm blanket at hand in case you get chilly. (Getting too cold can also make it hard for you to sleep.)

Keep it dark and quiet. A fan or a white-noise machine can muffle disturbing noises, and blackout shades or heavy drapes can block out light. You can also try earplugs and eyeshades.

Be careful about napping. Long naps can upset your sleeping schedule. If you're really exhausted, take a short nap in the afternoon, but avoid evening naps since they're too close to bedtime.

Exercise, but not too late in the day. You'll sleep better on the days you've exercised, but be aware that exercise increases your core body temperature for up to several hours. Finish your exercising at least a couple of hours before bedtime.

Avoid caffeine. Watch out for coffee, black tea, soft drinks, chocolate, and cocoa, or anything else containing caffeine. Some people find that drinking caffeine anytime after noon can interfere with their sleep.

Shun alcohol and heavy meals before bedtime. Although having a nightcap may sound like a good idea because of its relaxing effects, alcohol actually disrupts normal sleep patterns, triggers headaches, and makes early-morning awakenings more likely. Also, eating heavy meals too close to bedtime can keep your body in high gear as it tries to deal with all that food. Give yourself at least 2 hours to digest a big meal before you turn in for the night.

If you can't sleep, get up. If you've been lying in bed for half an hour and haven't dropped off to sleep, get up and do something mindless that doesn't require too much energy (like folding the laundry). When you feel really tired, go back to bed and try again. If you're still awake after 30 minutes, repeat the process. The idea is to keep from associating your bed with sleeplessness.

TRY THE HANDS-ON HEALING THERAPIES

The laying on of hands is one of the world's oldest healing arts and can be comforting, soothing, relaxing, and stimulating all at the same time. Massage, acupressure, and reflexology are just a few hands-on methods of relieving anxiety, irritability, and depression; increasing relaxation; lowering your heart rate and blood pressure; easing pain; and increasing your sense of well-being. Let's take a brief look at each to see how they can serve as effective, though temporary, anxiety busters.

Massage. Massage involves the manipulation of body tissues by stroking, rubbing, kneading, or exerting pressure, using the hands or instruments like rollers or pointers. There are many kinds of massage, but the one that is most effective for easing anxiety is Swedish massage. By kneading or stroking the muscles and putting pressure on tight, knotted muscles to break up tension, a massage therapist can relieve muscular stress and tension. As a bonus, massage increases circulation, improving the delivery of nutrients and oxygen to the cells.

Of course, you don't necessarily need to see a professional masseuse to reap these benefits. Ask your partner or a friend to give you a massage—then you can return the favor.

Acupressure. This soothing, relaxing hands-on therapy involves exerting pressure on various points throughout the body to break up energy blockages. According to traditional Chinese medicine theory, energy flows throughout the body courtesy of invisible channels called meridians. When one or more of these channels becomes blocked, the areas "downstream" of the blockage become painful or diseased. Luckily, the meridians run near the surface of the skin at some 300 points (called acupoints), and by exerting pressure on these points, blocked energy can be released.

To unblock the flow of energy and restore balance, the acupressurist uses the thumbs, fingers, whole hand, elbows, or feet, or tools such as balls, wooden rollers, and pointers.

Reflexology. This healing art involves applying pressure to certain reflex points on the soles of the feet, hands, and ears to increase relaxation, relieve pain, and encourage healing. All the glands, organs, and systems in the body are thought to be connected via nerves to a corresponding reflex point.

The reflexologist uses a map of the foot, hand, or ear to locate these points and then applies pressure using special thumb, finger, and hand techniques. Like acupressure, reflexology's goal is to break up energy blockages and bring the body back into balance.

To learn more about traditional massage, acupressure, and reflexology, see *The Book of Massage: The Complete Step-by-Step Guide to Eastern and Western Techniques,* by Lucinda Lidell, or check out our other suggested books in Recommended Reading and Resources on page 271.

THINK YOUR ANXIETY AWAY

Many of the cognitive-behavioral strategies we introduced in chapters 6 and 7—identifying and controlling cues, challenging Thought Myths, and rerouting your thinking—can also be applied to the irrational thoughts associated with anxiety.

For example, Judith noticed that every time she was getting ready to speak up in a PTA meeting, her heart would race and she would start to blush—before she even raised her hand. She realized that she had a Thought Myth in her head that said, "You're going to freeze and forget what you wanted to say, and everyone will stare at you." She challenged her Thought Myth and recalled that she did freeze once back in college (and was horrified) but also reminded herself that she has had many other situations in which people said she was an excellent speaker and expressed herself well. Then she decided, "So what if I blush? If I focus on it, it just gets worse." Reminding herself that the comments she wanted to make were for the good of her children, she rerouted her thought to be "I need to take deep breaths, stop focusing on my blushing, and think about the task at hand (instead of dwelling on my fears)."

STAND UP FOR YOURSELF!

If you have a problem with anxiety, give yourself permission to focus on your own needs for a change. You have the right to take care of your physical, mental, and emotional health. You have the right to pare down your responsibilities and your workload to a comfortable level. You have the right to have your needs, feelings, and rights recognized. You have the right to let others take responsibility for their own lives and actions. If you are the type of person who always gives 110 percent, you might want to try giving just 100 percent. Chances are that no one will notice the difference, and you can take some of the load off your shoulders. It's perfectly okay (and we encourage you) to do less and enjoy yourself more!

CHAPTER 10

Defuse Depression

Rachel's problem crept up on her so slowly that she didn't even realize anything was wrong. Feeling fatigued, she started sleeping more—going to bed earlier and getting up later. Since she worked at home as a writer, she could sneak naps during the day, a practice that became more and more attractive. Her business wasn't going well anyway, and for that matter, neither was her marriage.

Rachel would drink several cups of strong coffee to get herself jump-started in the morning. Then she'd sit at the computer for an hour or so, until her energy started to lag, prompting her to eat a couple of frozen waffles doused with syrup, after which she'd tumble back into bed for a nap.

Sometimes Rachel could get in a few good hours of work in the afternoon, but if she got frustrated or bored, she headed straight for the chocolate-marshmallow cookies, washing them down with a full-sugar soft drink. Then she often laid her head down on her desk and nodded off for 30 minutes or so. After a while, Rachel couldn't do anything but sleep the days away, getting up only long enough to eat something sweet or starchy before collapsing back into bed. Eventually, it dawned on her that she was suffering from depression, and a visit to her doctor confirmed her suspicion.

Depression is surprisingly common these days, with reported cases affecting about 9 percent of the population in any given 1-year period. It's an illness that has a particular affinity for females: Women are twice as likely as men to suffer from depression, a condition that affects more than 12 million adult females in the United States. The average age of onset is the late twenties, and women between the ages of 25 and 44 are more likely than anyone else to become depressed.

Why are women more likely to be depressed than men? Our reproductive biology, with its attendant shifts in hormones, plays a role. But genetics, work overload, family responsibilities, high levels of stress, the tendency to blame oneself, increased incidence of poverty, and higher rates of sexual abuse can all contribute to the high rates of depression seen among women. Luckily, depression can be improved in most women with the right treatment.

WHAT IS DEPRESSION?

Depression comes from the Latin word *deprimere,* which means a "pressing down." Indeed, it often feels like a heavy weight that's sitting squarely on top of your head or chest, and it strikes everyone occasionally. Feeling hopeless, helpless, or blue from time to time is a normal reaction to frustrating or difficult situations. For example, feeling sad, low in energy, or fatigued after you've experienced the loss of a job or the death of a loved one is natural. These feelings usually last for a finite period of time and eventually resolve themselves. Reflection, prayer, a talk with a close friend, time spent with the family, or a few visits to a psychologist or counselor can usually help ease this kind of depression.

But when the down feelings are stronger or last longer than one would expect in the situation, or depression strikes for no apparent reason, it's called major depressive disorder. This form of depression can result from an event that does not resolve, or it can appear to come out of the blue. Major depressive disorder should be taken seriously, with professional treatment sought. If your negative feelings linger for more than 2 weeks and you can't seem to find pleasure in the things you used to enjoy, you're probably suffering from a major depressive episode that requires treatment.

Are You Depressed?

Most people are well aware when they're depressed, as the signs are hard to miss: overwhelming feelings of sadness, grief, worthlessness, or hopelessness; inappropriate guilt; lack of motivation or low energy level; loss or gain of appetite; difficulty concentrating or making decisions; an agitated or antsy feeling; and changes in sleep patterns (either sleeping too much or too little). Sometimes people report that they don't feel anything at all—no pleasure and no sadness, just a sense of being flat. And not everyone experiences depression in terms of mood. Some people experience it in terms of physical symptoms, complaining of chronic headache, fatigue, weight loss or gain, decreased libido, or vague physical discomforts.

If you think that you are suffering from ongoing depression, even if it's a mild form, make an appointment to see your physician or a mental health professional right away. If you're not sure and you'd like to take a confidential depression screening test, visit the National Mental Health Association's depression screening Web site at www.depression-screening.org. You might also want to

MEDICATIONS AND DRUGS THAT CAN WORSEN DEPRESSION

The kinds of drugs listed below can trigger depression, make an existing depression worse, or both. If you're troubled by depression, it's essential that you stay away from alcohol and recreational drugs. And you may also want to consult your doctor about substituting other nondepressant medications for the prescription meds listed here.

- Alcohol
- Cocaine
- Estrogen
- High blood pressure medications
- Methamphetamines
- Opiates
- Steroids
- Tranquilizers (such as Ativan, Klonopin, Valium, and Xanax)

keep an eye out for National Depression Screening Day, a yearly event where health care providers educate the public about the symptoms of and effective treatments for depression, offer screening for depression, and help those in need to find treatment. To find the dates and locations of a depression screening site near you, log on to www.mentalhealthscreening.org/depression.htm.

WHAT TRIGGERS DEPRESSION?

Depression is the unhappy result of changes in both the body and the mind. Some people may be more likely to go through these changes because of early life experiences. Others may be genetically inclined toward depression or have endured a great many negative life events. Depression can also be caused by certain physical conditions or triggered by stressful or traumatic situations, but sometimes it just seems to appear out of nowhere. Many people are perplexed to find depression emerging just when things seemed to be going well in their lives.

Psychological factors. Stress can activate negative ideas about one's worth or competence that may have taken root in childhood or developed later in life. A person who had a critical, abusive, or unresponsive parent, for example, may have gotten the idea that she's incompetent or unlovable, ideas that will resurface later when something bad happens to her. She may end up blaming the negative event on herself because she feels inadequate or stupid.

Vulnerability to depression increases in people when they feel isolated or lacking in social support (for example, being in abusive relationships or raising children alone without help) or when they're under difficult social circumstances (such as enduring poverty, harassment, or job dissatisfaction). The thoughts one has when depressed often reflect a poor self-image, although depression really isn't about being inadequate or weak. It has more to do with the body and mind being overwhelmed and overstressed, which leaves one feeling helpless, hopeless, and exhausted.

Physical conditions. If you're depressed, it's important to determine whether an illness or physical condition is the cause. Visit your doctor to rule out the following:

- Anemia
- Cancer
- Central nervous system diseases
- Chronic infections
- Diabetes
- Hormonal imbalances, such as thyroid or adrenal disease
- Medication interactions
- Stroke
- Vitamin deficiency, such as a deficiency of B_{12}

In addition, depression during pregnancy and the postpartum period is not uncommon. Be sure to discuss your mental health, as well as your physical symptoms, during your regularly scheduled doctor visits.

Alterations in neurotransmitters. The brain is composed of trillions of nerve cells, with electrical messages rocketing through them at lightning speed. Many important types of nerve cells do not actually touch, so when a message is carried from one to another, it must be "ferried" across the gap between the two. Substances called neurotransmitters act as the "ferry." Three major neurotransmitters important for moods and emotions are dopamine, norepinephrine, and serotonin.

Scientists theorize that major depressive disorder results from changes in the amounts and functions of the neurotransmitters, alterations that destabilize the circuitry in the brain. The neurotransmitter that has received the most attention regarding both depression and problematic eating is serotonin, which has documented effects on mood, appetite regulation, and sleep. Most antidepressant medications—such as Prozac (fluoxetine), Zoloft (sertraline), and Paxil (paroxetine)—are aimed at normalizing serotonin function and increasing available amounts. Not surprisingly, many of these medications also influence appetite, weight gain, anxiety levels, and sleep.

SEROTONIN, DEPRESSION, AND RUNAWAY EATING

Serotonin is a powerful modulator of mood, appetite, pain awareness, and sleep. Although depression results from complex interplays among several neurotransmitters, low levels of serotonin in particular have been linked to a host of symptoms, including:

- Aggression and irritability
- Alcohol and drug abuse
- Anxiety
- Eating disorders, especially binge-eating and bulimia
- Increased sensitivity to pain
- Low mood
- Mania and mood swings
- Migraines
- Obsessive-compulsive disorder
- Premenstrual syndrome (PMS), particularly food cravings and moodiness
- Seasonal affective disorder (SAD)
- Sleep disorders, especially insomnia

Because all these symptoms have low serotonin levels in common, they often appear in clusters. For example, people with bulimia nervosa tend to have higher rates of depression, anxiety, and substance abuse than people without bulimia. Those who suffer from depression have a greater tendency toward alcohol abuse and migraines than those who aren't depressed, and those with insomnia tend to be more anxious than those who sleep well. Although serotonin certainly isn't the only neurotransmitter that influences mood, sleep, appetite, and substance abuse, it does play a major role.

Serotonin's Role in Appetite, Bingeing, and Restricting

Depression almost always goes hand in hand with appetite changes—some depressed people stop eating or eat very little, and others eat more than usual. The appetite-depression link is so clear cut, in fact, that unexplained weight loss or gain is considered a diagnostic sign of depression.

Serotonin may be the culprit behind both problems. Research confirms that serotonin levels tend to be below normal in women with active bulimia nervosa, and that reduced serotonin levels are related to an increase in appetite and overeating in both animals and humans. In a study of bulimic patients, for example, depletion of tryptophan, the "raw material" from which serotonin is made, corresponded with an increase in the size of the meals the patients ate. Conversely, when serotonin availability or activity was regulated, appetite and food consumption normalized. Serotonin levels may also increase in response to bingeing or bingeing and purging, possibly assisting with improving mood, energy, and concentration.

On the other hand, high levels of serotonin activity in the brain are associated with appetite suppression, food restriction, anxiety, and obsessive behaviors, all of which are characteristic of

SEROTONIN AND RUNAWAY EATING

Abnormal levels of serotonin can bring about the following symptoms, all of which play a part in Runaway Eating.

- High levels of anxiety and nervousness
- Rigid behaviors (thinking there is only one right way to do things)
- Ritualistic behaviors (doing things in a certain way all the time)
- Obsessive thoughts and behaviors (thinking or doing the same thing over and over again)
- Decreased or increased appetite
- Impulsivity
- Moodiness or irritability
- Low or sad mood
- Low energy
- Poor concentration

anorexia. By restricting food intake, the amount of available serotonin can be decreased, which may also decrease the anxiety and obsessive behavior. So without even knowing it, people with eating disorders and Runaway Eating may be trying to regulate their abnormal serotonin levels through their eating habits.

The Effects of Carbs on Serotonin Levels

Carbohydrate consumption plays an important part in determining how much serotonin your body makes, so it's no coincidence that typical binge foods—ice cream, cake, candy, cookies, bread, and even mashed potatoes—tend to be very high in carbs such as sugar and starch. Serotonin is synthesized within the brain from tryptophan, an amino acid found primarily in animal protein. But the tryptophan can't reach the brain without first hitching a ride on a carrier molecule. Several other amino acids also need to hitch rides on the same kind of carrier molecule, so there's a lot of competition. The tryptophan often gets left out and doesn't make it to the brain, which means that less serotonin is produced. But thanks to carbohydrates, tryptophan can go to the front of the line and hop onto carrier molecules before the other amino acids, allowing it to enter the brain more readily. That's because carbohydrates trigger the release of insulin, which rounds up the other circulating amino acids and takes them off to make protein. In effect, the insulin temporarily removes tryptophan's competition, making it much easier for tryptophan to hop onto a carrier molecule and travel to the brain. The result is a higher concentration of tryptophan in the brain, which can then be converted into more serotonin. So there's a reason that you automatically head for the cookies or the chocolate cake when you're feeling down. Your body may be trying to raise its serotonin levels.

LOW-CARB DIETS AND DEPRESSION

Low-carb/high-protein diets are currently all the rage—even fast-food restaurants have added "bunless burgers" and low-carb cookies to their menus. But if you tend toward Runaway Eating, and especially if you struggle with depression, following a low-carb diet could be particularly detrimental. That's because cutting back on carbs may have unfavorable effects on your serotonin levels. Low serotonin can influence your mood and even increase negative thinking, both of which do much to keep the Runaway Eating cycle in motion.

Bad moods. As described earlier, in order for serotonin to be produced, tryptophan must first hitch a ride into the brain. Foods that are low in protein and high in carbohydrates trigger the release of insulin, which takes away the amino acids that compete with tryptophan for a "seat" on a carrier molecule. But in order for this to work, you need to eat a meal or snack high in carbs and low in protein.

Of course, low-carb diets contain exactly the opposite combination: foods high in protein and low in carbohydrates. High-protein diets have been shown to depress tryptophan levels, because the amino acids competing with tryptophan return in force. This could lead to lower amounts of tryptophan making its way to the brain, which could be bad news if you already produce too little serotonin. So low-carb diets may be double trouble for some people: They result in very little "raw material" getting to the brain for serotonin production, and the high-protein foods eaten with virtually every meal or snack may block the serotonin-promoting capabilities of the carbs that are eaten. If low levels of serotonin result, they may lead to feelings of depression, anxiety, irritability, tension, and fatigue—all well-established triggers of Runaway Eating.

Negative thinking. Whether you're following a strict low-carb diet plan or just trying to stay away from carbs as much as possible, one thing is for certain: You're on a *diet,* and diets are major promoters of Runaway Eating. Like all other diets, the low-carb version encourages rigid, hypercontrolled behavior, all-or-nothing thinking, the idea of "good foods/bad foods," obsessive thoughts and behaviors about eating, and interference with the body's natural hunger and fullness signals. And, because it is a diet that you can go on and off, chances are good that you'll eventually blow it, triggering feelings of failure, depression, and self-loathing, all of which increase Runaway Eating.

NATURAL STRATEGIES TO EASE DEPRESSION—AND RUNAWAY EATING

If necessary, your doctor can prescribe medications to treat depression that may also help treat Runaway Eating. But there are also several effective natural methods of combating depression, including cognitive-behavioral skills, exercise, diet, and light therapy. Let's take a closer look at each method.

Cognitive-Behavioral Skills

Although we showed you in chapters 6 and 7 how to use cognitive-behavioral therapy (CBT) as a tool to treat Runaway Eating, it was first developed as a treatment for depression. Aaron T. Beck, M.D., the founder of cognitive-behavioral therapy, professor of psychiatry at the University of Pennsylvania School of Medicine in Philadelphia, and coauthor of the seminal book *Cognitive Therapy of Depression,* recognized that negative thoughts about one's self, the world, and the future could cause and perpetuate a depressed mood. He urged patients to identify these negative thoughts and replace them with healthier alternatives.

The beauty of cognitive-behavioral therapy tools is that they can help in many problem areas. Take a look at the example below, to see how CBT can be applied to depressive thoughts.

Susan, a highly successful graphic designer, was troubled from time to time by depressed moods that seemed to come out of nowhere and take over her life. Suddenly her self-confidence would plummet; she'd lose all perspective and start doubting her own considerable abilities. Before she knew it, she'd be caught in a whirlpool of negative thoughts that pulled her further and further into depression. Needless to say, these low moods made it especially difficult for Susan to come up with creative ideas and do her job well.

After going through a course of cognitive-behavioral therapy, Susan began to recognize these negative and self-defeating thoughts when they appeared. Then she used her CBT tools to get herself back on track before the negative thoughts got the best of her. When the low moods descended, Susan referred to the following list of thoughts, ideas, and actions that could help get her through the day, a day at a time (sometimes an hour at a time), until her mood lifted again.

1. I realize that my thoughts are distorted right now and are part of the depression, rather than a reflection of who I am.
2. I will break my tasks down into smaller, more manageable chunks and give myself a mental reward whenever I get through one of them.

3. I know that this mood will eventually pass. If I just use my CBT tools, I'll start to experience some relief before long.
4. I will reach out to my friends and occasionally call my old therapist for a booster session or two.
5. I will make time for exercise every day.
6. I will not skip meals, shortchange myself on sleep, or drown my mood in alcohol.
7. I will allow myself to get lost in a movie or a good book to get my mind off my worries.

Although sometimes it could take a week or so before Susan realized that her mood was slipping and she was sinking into negative thinking, once she caught on, she could usually get hold of her thoughts fairly quickly and avoid sinking into a major depressive episode.

To use cognitive-behavioral therapy to combat your own low mood or depressive thoughts, turn back to chapters 6 and 7 and try the strategies listed there to derail negative thoughts and replace them with healthier ones.

Exercise: A Natural Serotonin Booster

Regular exercise is a natural antidepressant that can do much to improve your mood. It helps release stress, relax the muscles, improve alertness and concentration by boosting the oxygen supply to the brain, reduce insomnia, and stimulate the production of endorphins, neurotransmitters that increase the feeling of well-being. It may also improve your outlook on life. Australian researchers found that long-term exercisers think more positively and feel more positive about their day-to-day experiences than nonexercisers or short-term exercisers.

It appears that exercise—particularly rhythmic exercises and repetitive activities—may also help regulate serotonin function. Studies performed by Barry Jacobs, Ph.D., of the Princeton University program in neuroscience reveal a connection between movement and the activity of serotonin. In animal tests, he found that serotonin action was at its highest during the most active parts of the day and lowest during REM sleep, when the body becomes temporarily paralyzed. Rhythmic, repetitive movements appeared to increase serotonin system activity markedly.

Of course, if you're depressed, often the last thing you want to do is get up and exercise. It's easier if you have an already-established exercise routine that you do rain or shine, no matter how you feel. It also helps to make your session as enjoyable as possible. Some people find it easier to exercise as part of a class. Pick an activity that's pleasurable for you, try to incorporate some music if you can, and vary your routine so that you don't get bored. And don't forget to reward yourself in a nonfood way after you've finished.

Diet: Finding the Right Balance of Carbs and Protein for You

The eating plan we recommended in chapter 5 is based on solid nutritional information and is designed to provide the body with sufficient nutrients and help regulate blood sugar levels. However, if you're having problems with bingeing (or urges to binge), anxiety, or depression, all of which may be related to low serotonin levels, you might want to try the following experiment for a few days.

For the first 2 days, eat according to the suggestions outlined in chapter 5, which means that all your meals and snacks will include carbohydrates and protein. Use your "Daily Logs for Self-Monitoring" throughout the day to record everything you eat, your moods, levels of hunger, and urges to binge. Then, for the next 2 days, substitute a serving of carbohydrates for the protein both in your breakfast and in your afternoon snack. That is, eat a slice of bread, some whole grain cereal, a fruit, or a vegetable instead of the protein-containing food (including milk) that you would normally have. Both your breakfast and afternoon snack will now consist of higher proportions of carbohydrates relative to protein. Eat your other meals as suggested in the food plan in chapter 5 and add the protein that you would have eaten at breakfast and at snack time to your other meals. Again, record everything you eat, your moods, levels of hunger, and urges to binge.

The idea is to see if varying the carbohydrate-protein ratio in these meals has an impact on your mood and urges to binge. The rationale behind the experiment comes from a study with humans that showed that a carbohydrate-rich breakfast significantly increases the amount of tryptophan in the blood, but a protein-rich breakfast has no such effect. Although the amount of tryptophan in the blood doesn't necessarily mean that more serotonin will be produced in the brain, it is a possibility.

If you find that eating the carbohydrate-rich breakfast or snack increases your hunger or urge to binge, makes you feel light-headed, shaky, or just plain worse, stop the experiment and go back to the original eating plan. But if you find that you feel better, less hungry, or less inclined to binge, eating a high-carbohydrate, low-protein breakfast and afternoon snack may be something you want to do regularly. However, under no circumstances should you stop eating protein altogether—or even cut back on the recommended daily amounts.

Light Therapy

You may not be aware of it, but your exposure to light affects your emotional health to a remarkable degree. Most people experience a slight dip in mood (or at least a little regret) when they have to turn their clocks back in autumn, and darkness falls in the late afternoon. But some of us experience more-extreme symptoms when the days grow shorter. These may include depression or a worsening of problems like alcohol abuse or dependence, bipolar disorder, PMS, bulimia nervosa, and sleep disorders. This is especially common in northerly areas like Alaska, where light is scarce for months at a time. But why would light make a difference in your mood?

Light and darkness play crucial roles in the sleep cycle and, ultimately, in mood. When the sun goes down or you're in a dark, dimly lit area, your pineal gland begins to produce high levels of melatonin, a hormone that helps you shift into low gear, become drowsy, and get ready for sleep. In the morning, when you are exposed to bright light, your melatonin levels recede, waking you up, increasing your energy and concentration, and getting you ready to face the day. But until you are exposed to bright light, your melatonin levels tend to stay high, keeping you sleepy and lethargic. High levels of melatonin are a major reason that it's so hard to get up when it's still dark outside, or why we feel like rushing home and getting into bed when darkness falls at 5:00 P.M.

Many people suffer from seasonal affective disorder (SAD), a form of depression that recurs each year during the fall and winter. The farther north you go, the higher the rates of SAD. The lack of exposure to bright light during these seasons can make those who are sensitive to melatonin feel apathetic, lethargic, depressed, anxious, or sleepy. They also often crave carbohydrates (or sweets), which can lead to weight gain.

If you suspect your mood is sensitive to the light/dark cycle, you can help yourself by getting plenty of full-spectrum light. The Scandinavians are well aware of this phenomenon. As the dark winter months approach, they start to flock to light cafés in order to increase their exposure to full-spectrum light. Full-spectrum light comes from two sources—sunlight and special full-spectrum lightbulbs—and contains all the wavelengths of sunlight. The regular incandescent or fluorescent lights that we typically find in our homes and offices are not effective at treating depression.

Getting more full-spectrum light is easy—just take a 10-minute walk in bright sunlight every day, preferably first thing in the morning. And if it's cloudy? Don't worry—you can still absorb some full-spectrum light, so try to get outside for a while despite the overcast weather. Don't wear your glasses (unless you absolutely have to), sunglasses, or tinted contacts, because they will block some of the wavelengths.

If you live in a northerly area that has short days and little sun, try replacing your incandescent lightbulbs (the kind used in most lamps) with full-spectrum lightbulbs. Vita-Lite bulbs, which are used to light indoor gardens, provide full-spectrum light and are available in some nurseries and hardware stores. Simply changing your lightbulbs may be enough to ease your depression, but if it isn't, consider buying a special full-spectrum light box. The light is measured in units called lux, and it takes at least 2,500 lux to exert a therapeutic effect on depression. Daylight provides about 5,000 lux; the typical light box provides 10,000 lux.

You can find a selection of light boxes at most medical supply stores or through a host of Internet suppliers (just go to a search

(continued on page 202)

NATURAL DEPRESSION RELIEVERS

Certain natural supplements have shown promise as depression relievers. Though more research is needed to confirm their effectiveness and overall safety, you may want to talk with your doctor to see if any might be right for you. Be aware that combining these substances with a prescription antidepressant can be dangerous or deadly, so exercise caution and use these substances only in consultation with your physician.

DLPA. A form of the amino acid phenylalanine, DLPA is believed to help ease depression by protecting against the destruction of endorphins, naturally occurring substances in the body that block pain and help regulate mood. Low endorphin levels have been linked to chronic pain and depression, and some studies have shown that DLPA can help with both of these conditions.

■ In one study, 40 patients with major depression were given DLPA plus vitamin B$_6$ twice daily. Thirty-one of the 40 improved "almost immediately," and 10 of these 31 were completely relieved of depression.

■ Twenty-three depressed people, who had not been helped by medications, were given phenylalanine. Two weeks later, 17 of 23 had no symptoms of depression.

■ DLPA was given to 370 depressed patients. Fifteen days later, 73 percent enjoyed a "normal affective state." And 1½ months later, that number had risen to 80 percent, and another 15 percent showed some improvement.

Typical doses of DLPA start at 350 milligrams twice a day for a person who weighs at least 110 pounds. Those who weigh less should take a little less. Because DLPA protects endorphins rather than producing them, it takes a while (up to 2 weeks) for enough endorphins to accumulate to combat depression.

Caution: Some people, including those with phenylketonuria (PKU) or alkaptonuria, cannot metabolize phenylalanine properly and should not take DLPA. Those on a phenylalanine-restricted diet should also avoid the supplement. Combining phenylalanine with monoamine oxidase inhibitors, Eldepryl (selegiline), levodopa, and neuroleptic drugs may be dangerous. If you have hypertension, stroke, schizophrenia, or tyrosinemia/tyrosinuria, you should take DLPA only under your physician's supervision.

Omega-3 fatty acids. One study of the effect of omega-3 fatty acids (the kind of fat found in cold-water fatty fish) on patients with bipolar disorder (manic depression) found that taking large amounts in supplement form helped to stabilize their condition. And lower levels of aggression were seen in stressed-out students taking final examinations who took omega-3 supplements.

Although there is no established dose of omega-3 fatty acids, 1 to 3 grams is typical.

Caution: Fish oil can interfere with medications that have anticoagulant or antiplatelet actions and increase the risk of bleeding. It can also interfere with certain antidiabetic and antihypertensive drugs. Use with caution if you have hypertension, diabetes, or cirrhosis, or are aspirin sensitive. Consult your physician before taking fish oil.

5-HTP. As tryptophan is the raw material from which serotonin is made, it may make sense to go to the source and take tryptophan in supplement form. The FDA-approved form of the amino acid is 5-hydroxytryptophan (5-HTP, for short).

You may remember that tryptophan supplements were banned in the late 1980s when a tainted batch imported from Japan caused some serious reactions, including several deaths. This form of the amino acid has since been declared illegal in the United States, even though the supplement itself was never proven to be a danger. 5-HTP is a related form but isn't exactly the same.

Studies have shown that taking 5-HTP boosts tryptophan levels in the brain, although it hasn't yet been proven to increase serotonin levels. Still, several studies have produced encouraging results.

- 5-HTP taken alone or combined with another substance in a Swiss study of depression treatments on 25 patients proved to be just as effective at

(continued)

relieving depression as were traditional antidepressants.

- A 2002 review of published studies using 5-HTP or tryptophan for treatment of depression found that both are effective for relieving depression. The survey was performed by the Cochrane Database, a highly respected reviewer of medical literature.

Caution: Side effects associated with large amounts of 5-HTP include loss of appetite, diarrhea, nausea, and vomiting. Some reports have associated 5-HTP with blood disorders. Consult your physician before using 5-HTP with medications such as carbidopa and serotonin agonists.

SAMe. A naturally occurring substance with the tongue-twisting formal name of S-adenosyl-L-methionine, SAMe is derived from the amino acid methionine. Its multiple duties in the body include aiding in the manufacture of hormones, neurotransmitters, and proteins, as well as protecting against mutation of DNA. In pharmacological doses of up to 1 gram a day, SAMe may help reduce depression by spurring the body's production of serotonin.

- From Italy come two studies that tested whether or not SAMe can help relieve the symptoms of major depressive disorder. In one trial, participants were given either the drug imipramine (a standard antidepressant) or injections of SAMe. In the other, they received either imipramine or an oral dose of SAMe. Whether oral or injectable, SAMe was found to be just as effective as the drug at relieving depression, with fewer side effects.
- In a larger study done in 2002, injections of SAMe were compared with injections of imipramine. Two hundred and ninety-three people suffering from major depression participated. Half received the SAMe injections for about a month, and the other half, the drug. SAMe proved to be just as effective as the drug but with fewer side effects.

Caution: SAMe does have side effects, including nausea, headaches, anxiety, mania, and hypomania. The higher the dose, the greater the risk of side effects. SAMe should not be used while you are taking antidepressants.

St. John's wort *(Hypericum perforatum).* In Germany, St. John's wort is widely prescribed for depression, and many studies have shown that it is effective. Some people believe that St. John's wort helps control serotonin levels in the brain, but researchers have not definitively proved this. We do know that this herb helps ease the symptoms of depression in many people through its muscle-relaxing and mild tranquilizing properties.

- German researchers found that an extract of St. John's wort was just as effective as imipramine in treating 324 people with mild to moderate depression—but the herb caused fewer side effects.
- From the *British Medical Journal* comes a report of a study with 263 people in which St. John's wort was compared with imipramine and a placebo. St. John's wort was found to be more effective than the placebo and at least as effective as the medication.

Caution: Though St. John's wort extract has been widely used in Germany with no reports of serious problems with toxicity or long-term usage, the herb's side effects including fatigue, headache, insomnia, and restlessness. It may be dangerous to combine St. John's wort with other herbs that have sedative properties, antidepressants, oral contraceptives, narcotics, warfarin, or other drugs. Combining this herb with a selective serotonin reuptake inhibitor or a monoamine oxidase inhibitor can be dangerous or deadly. In some cases, St. John's wort may actually worsen major depressive disorder, bipolar disorder, and infertility. Let your physician know about all the supplements you're taking, and consult your physician before beginning any regimen that includes herbs.

engine and type in "light box" to find them). Prices range from $200 to $500, but if the box is prescribed by a doctor, your insurance company may cover at least part of the cost.

Once a day, turn on the light box, face it (but don't look directly at the light), and sit in front of it for a period of 15 to 45 minutes, beginning at the lower end of the range and working your way up. You may read, write, eat, talk on the phone, or do anything else you want while you receive the light therapy, but don't close your eyes or wear tinted glasses or tinted contacts.

For most people, it's best to receive light therapy first thing in the morning (before 8:00 A.M.). Light therapy later in the evening or before bedtime may make it more difficult to fall asleep.

Caution: The side effects of light therapy can include eyestrain, red eyes, fatigue, headaches, irritability, or an inability to sleep (which is usually due to evening light therapy). If any of these arise, either limit your exposure or stop the therapy. Consult your doctor before trying light therapy if your eyes or skin are light sensitive or if you're taking antibiotics, antipsychotic drugs, or medication for psoriasis or vitiligo. Do not use the light box when you're feeling manic or hyperactive.

MORE STRATEGIES TO EASE DEPRESSION

Many of the techniques we've discussed in chapters 6 through 8 (such as using relaxation techniques and simplifying your life) are also helpful for easing depression. In addition, consider these ideas for warding off depression before it sets in.

Avoid alcohol. Alcohol is a depressant that works directly on the central nervous system, so anyone with depression should avoid it. Alcohol is derived from sugar, so it promotes a rise and fall in blood sugar that heightens anxiety, irritability, anger, and bad moods. It also depletes the body of substantial amounts of B vitamins, vitamin C, calcium, magnesium, potassium, and zinc, which can lead to deficiency-induced depression. The less alcohol you drink, the better.

Limit caffeine. Caffeine gives you a lift, but it also stimulates a release of insulin that can clear too much glucose from your bloodstream, leaving you weak, hungry, craving sweets, and depressed. Too much caffeine can also induce anxiety-like symptoms. If you must have caffeine-containing beverages, limit your intake to one or two per day and drink them as part of a meal. If you are prone to insomnia, either give up caffeine entirely or stay away from it in the afternoon and evening.

Get plenty of B vitamins. It's long been established that the B vitamins are linked to mood. A major reason is the critical role they play in manufacturing neurotransmitters. Deficiencies in B vitamins can translate to lower levels of these vital brain chemicals, which can affect mood and behavior.

For example, a lack of thiamin (B_1) can cause mental confusion, emotional instability, depression, and irritability. Deficiencies in riboflavin (B_2)—which affect as many as one-quarter of elderly patients suffering from depression—can bring on depression, lethargy, and fatigue. Too little niacin (B_3) can cause depression, irritability, and insomnia. Vitamin B_6 plays a vital role in the production of serotonin, so if it's lacking, a depression resulting from low serotonin levels can ensue. Even small deficiencies in B_{12} increase the risk of depression, memory loss, and paranoia. And a shortage of folic acid is often found in depressed patients, most likely because it lowers levels of both serotonin and SAMe (S-adenosyl-L-methionine) in the brain.

Correcting B-vitamin deficiencies has alleviated or at least eased depression in many cases. Boosting thiamin levels was found to lift the mood of participants in at least four different double-blind studies. Vitamin B_6 supplementation has been shown to stabilize the mood in suicidal or depressed patients with low neurotransmitter levels. Folic acid supplements given to patients who were depressed and lacking in this vitamin helped them recover faster. And vitamin B_{12} supplements improved mood and memory in patients who had mental illness related to a B_{12} deficiency.

The B vitamins are found in a variety of foods, including avocados, bananas, beans, broccoli, brown rice, cauliflower, chicken breast, dried sunflower seeds, fish, orange juice, peanuts, spinach, and wheat germ. Be sure to include plenty of these foods in your diet.

As for supplements, be aware that the B vitamins are part of a "family," and they work best when all family members are present. Don't take a supplement that supplies just one or two of the Bs. A balanced B supplement will contain thiamin, riboflavin, niacin, B_6, B_{12}, pantothenic acid, and folic acid. Most multivitamin/mineral products have a B complex as part of the formula, so if you take a multivitamin that provides 100 percent of the Daily Value for each of the B vitamins, you're probably well covered.

Get professional help if necessary. Depression should be taken seriously. If you don't get relief after trying some of the techniques in this chapter, you feel your depression worsening, you just don't have the motivation to help yourself, or you find yourself becoming suicidal, consult a mental health professional. Or speak to your primary care provider, who can steer you in the right direction. Although many milder forms of depression respond well to the self-help approaches described in this chapter, more-severe depression may require medication, face-to-face psychotherapy, and careful monitoring by a mental health professional.

CHAPTER 11

Manage Menopausal Symptoms

Being a woman is a dramatic thing. Your body, mind, and emotions go through myriad changes as you navigate the high seas of puberty and the hormonal changes of your monthly cycle. If you have a child, the changes you experience during pregnancy, delivery, breastfeeding, and the postpartum period may leave you baffled—but in awe. Yet of all the hormonal upheavals that occur throughout a lifetime, many women find that those experienced during midlife rival any they have ever known.

Many people think that menopause is a long, drawn-out process that can go on for several years. But the term, which is derived from the Greek words *men* ("month") and *pausis* ("end"), actually refers to a single event, the moment when your last period has ended. Menopause is part of a much longer process called the climacteric, during which your ovaries stop releasing eggs, and levels of your female hormones fluctuate wildly and gradually decline. Believe it or not, the climacteric begins way back when you're in your late twenties or early thirties and continues over a period of 35 years or longer, coming to a close in your late fifties or early sixties, when your hormones finally stabilize at low but constant levels. Most women experience menopause around the age of 50, although it may occur as early as your thirties or, rarely, as late as your late fifties.

THE LINK BETWEEN MENOPAUSE AND RUNAWAY EATING

As your female hormones fluctuate and gradually decrease during the 4 to 10 years preceding your last menstrual period (a phase known as perimenopause) and for a couple of years afterward, the delicate balance that exists between these hormones can be thrown for a loop. In some women, this causes intense changes in mood, appetite, sleeping patterns, body shape, and weight. Often it's unclear which changes are due to menopause and which are just part of the aging process, and at first they may be so subtle that you don't even notice them. But somewhere between the ages of 35 and 45, as your hormone levels become more erratic, you'll definitely see and feel the difference.

Your periods will become irregular and may be lighter or heavier than usual. You may skip your period for a month or two, or you may get it twice in 1 month. Your mood can begin to suffer, and you may find yourself more prone to irritability and fatigue. A problem with insomnia or early-morning awakening can suddenly arise, leaving you tired, anxious, and hypersensitive. Hot flashes and night sweats can leave you uncomfortable, drenched in sweat, and tired from the sleep disturbances they cause. Your glucose tolerance can lessen, bringing on sugar cravings, bingeing, mood swings, and fatigue. You may also develop a problem with water retention, making you feel fat and bloated. To make matters worse, your metabolism may begin to slow, and you may gain weight more easily, especially around the middle, even though your eating habits haven't changed.

Feeling fat, bloated, tired, anxious, and depressed, you're much more likely to fall into Runaway Eating behaviors during this time, especially if you're already inclined in that direction. In short, if you want to protect yourself from Runaway Eating, you'll need to take charge of your menopausal symptoms. The good news is that there are many strategies you can try that will help ease your symptoms and keep Runaway Eating at bay.

THE MAGICAL MENSTRUAL CYCLE

Before we talk about the "solution," we need to lay out the problem. And to understand the challenges, we need to know how things work during a normal menstrual cycle, when all the elements are working together in perfect harmony.

Estrogen Plays the Starring Role, at Least in the Beginning

We begin with Day 1, which is the first day of menstruation. Within the first few days of the cycle, a control center in the brain, known as the hypothalamus, signals the pituitary gland that it's time to get some eggs ready for fertilization.

The pituitary gland then produces follicle-stimulating hormone (FSH) and luteinizing hormone (LH). FSH triggers the production of estrogen, and anywhere from 3 to 30 of the eggs residing in the ovaries begin to grow. Each egg is encased in a protective wrapper called a follicle, a casing that does double duty as a hormone factory. As the eggs grow, the follicles increase in size as well and begin to produce their own supply of estrogen.

During the first half of the menstrual cycle (approximately the first 14 days), estrogen is the dominant hormone, and levels of it continue to increase. It makes the lining of the uterus thick and causes blood vessels in the uterine wall to grow. This creates a hospitable, nutrient-rich place for a fertilized egg to lodge. The follicles continue to grow larger, producing more and more estrogen, until one of them proves to be the largest and most fit. This will be the one to produce this month's egg.

At the same time, LH and FSH levels have slowly begun to climb. Then around Day 13 of the cycle, when estrogen levels climax with a surge of their most potent version, estradiol, LH and FSH levels also climb. They both peak on Day 14, prompting the ripened egg to blast out of its follicle (a process called ovulation). The egg is finally free to float through the Fallopian tube toward the uterus, toward a possible union with a sperm cell. But we're only halfway through the story. . . .

Progesterone Takes Center Stage

Once the egg bursts out of its old house, the follicle, and starts on its journey, you might think that the follicle would simply disintegrate and be reabsorbed by the body. Instead, the follicle takes on a completely new identity, transforming itself into a potent hormone factory called the corpus luteum.

While the corpus luteum continues to produce estrogen, it adds an important new ingredient to the mix—large amounts of progesterone, which is the dominant hormone during the last half of the menstrual cycle. As progesterone levels rise, the lining of the uterus becomes spongy and even more hospitable to the fertilized egg. Progesterone builds toward a climax, and estrogen heads for its second peak, with both reaching a crescendo at about Day 23. Then, if the egg hasn't been fertilized and implanted in the uterine wall, both of these hormones rapidly drop down to nearly nothing, the thickened lining of the uterus breaks down, and within about 5 days the lining begins to shed, starting Day 1 of a new menstrual cycle.

ESTROGEN AND PROGESTERONE: A BALANCING ACT

Estrogen and progesterone, the star hormones of the female reproductive system, exist in a delicate balance. On the one hand, they oppose and counterbalance each other, like two children on a seesaw, to make sure that neither one exerts more influence than it should. But on the other hand, each sensitizes receptors for the other throughout the body. So progesterone helps the body take up estrogen, and estrogen helps the body take up progesterone.

Estrogen encourages the body to deposit fat in certain areas (particularly the breasts, hips, and thighs), which contributes to the curviness of the female form. It also spurs retention of salt and fluid, promotes cell growth, builds up the uterine lining, and increases blood clotting. All of these are necessary when preparing the body for impending motherhood.

Progesterone does the opposite. Estrogen builds up the uterine lining, then progesterone helps break the lining down and shed it. Estrogen promotes deposition of body fat, then progesterone spurs the body to break down the fat and use it for energy. And estrogen increases the clotting of the blood, then progesterone helps normalize it. Working together, the estrogen-progesterone system of checks and balances keeps the reproductive system and several other bodily functions working in harmony.

Perimenopause and Estrogen Dominance

During perimenopause, the harmony that had existed between estrogen and progesterone can change to discord. Even though you may continue to have regular menstrual periods, there will be months when no egg is produced. And when there's no egg, there's no corpus luteum (the discarded "wrapper" on the egg) to manufacture progesterone. During these months, your progesterone levels will fall nearly to zero, although your estrogen levels may continue along on their normal course. This throws the body into a state of estrogen dominance, in which estrogen is allowed to exert its effects without the balancing influence of progesterone.

What does this mean for you? For starters, because estrogen promotes water retention, without progesterone's counterbalancing effects, you may experience bloating, weight gain, breast tenderness, and tissue swelling. Too much estrogen can also bring on low blood sugar, a diminished sex drive, depression, and magnesium deficiency, which can trigger sugar cravings and mood swings.

Not only is estrogen dominance a major factor during the years just preceding menopause, it's also a prime factor in PMS. It can result from poor diet, too much body fat (fatty tissue produces estrogen), stress, oral contraceptives, estrogen-only hormone replacement therapy, or liver dysfunction. Additional symptoms of estrogen dominance include:

- Anxiety
- Breast tenderness
- Cravings (especially for sugar, caffeine, and carbohydrates)
- Depression
- Emotional hypersensitivity

- Fatigue
- Headaches, including migraines
- Hypoglycemia (low blood sugar)
- Insomnia
- Irritability
- Low sex drive
- Moodiness
- Slow thyroid
- Uterine fibroids
- Water retention
- Weight gain

Menopause and Dwindling Estrogen

Estrogen excess is common during the years before the last menstrual period, but once you segue into menopause and postmenopause, a more pressing problem may be dwindling estrogen levels. The most obvious sign of low estrogen is the cessation of your menstrual cycle, which many women consider a benefit after years of painful or inconvenient periods. But the loss of this important hormone carries with it a host of detriments and can wield a mighty punch physically, mentally, and emotionally.

Because estrogen receptors are sprinkled throughout the central nervous system, too little of this hormone can wreak havoc on your emotional and mental states. Pronounced mood fluctuations, moodiness, irritability, increasing forgetfulness, and fuzzy thinking are reported by some women during the menopausal years. The risk of cardiovascular disease rises sharply, because lowered levels of estrogen increase both total cholesterol and the "bad" LDL cholesterol, while decreasing the "good" HDL cholesterol. Blood pressure rises, and the rate at which plaque is deposited inside the arteries increases, making strokes and heart attacks more likely. Too little estrogen is also directly related to the development of osteoporosis, or thinning of the bones, a major cause of disability and even death in women over 50.

By far the most common complaint related to low levels of estrogen is hot flashes; about 85 percent of all women in the United States experience them. Hot flashes—waves of heat that spread upward toward your face and down your shoulders—ratchet up your blood pressure and heart rate. The blood vessels dilate, and the sweat pores open wide, leaving you drenched in perspiration. Night sweats are the nocturnal version of hot flashes and can cause middle-of-the-night awakenings and a decrease in dreamtime (REM) sleep, contributing to insomnia and daytime fatigue. Other conditions related to too little estrogen include:

- Anxiety
- Bladder infections
- Cardiovascular disease
- Cessation of the menstrual cycle
- Depression
- Forgetfulness
- Hot flashes/night sweats
- Insomnia
- Irregular menstrual cycles
- Irritability
- Lack of concentration
- Mood swings
- Osteoporosis
- Urinary incontinence
- Vaginal dryness and thinning
- Vaginal infections

Luckily, almost nobody suffers from all of these problems! And some of them—most notably hot flashes, night sweats, insomnia, and emotional changes—are temporary. But others, like high blood pressure, high cholesterol, atherosclerosis, and osteoporosis, can pose serious threats to your health. Although for the past 3 decades the medical community has promoted hormone replacement therapy as the one-size-fits-all solution, the results of recent long-term, large-scale studies show that this isn't the answer. Fortunately, there are many lifestyle changes and natural approaches to balancing your hormones and easing menopausal symptoms that work quite well and have few to no side effects. In the rest of this chapter, we'll take a look at natural ways to alleviate the menopausal symptoms that can trigger Runaway Eating.

TACKLING MENOPAUSE SYMPTOMS WITH NUTRITIONAL AND LIFESTYLE CHANGES

Two of the most common menopausal symptoms are anxiety and the fatigue caused by interrupted sleep. For natural solutions for both of these, turn back to chapter 9. Also, chapter 10 offers numerous strategies for handling depression, a common menopausal symptom. Of the menopausal symptoms that are left, the four that are most likely to encourage unhealthy eating behaviors are menopause-related weight gain, appetite changes, blood sugar imbalances, and water retention.

Menopause-Related Weight Gain

At the onset of menopause, you may find both your weight and your waistline increasing, even if your eating habits haven't changed. And it's not your imagination—an increase in obesity and a change in fat distribution that favors the abdominal area are common during menopause. The weight gain is probably largely due to decreases in activity and the age-related slowing down of your metabolism, but declining estrogen also contributes to the problem. It causes an increase in fatty tissue compared with lean body tissue and ensures that any weight you may gain in the future will have a higher fat content than before. The tendency for fat to settle around your middle—as it does in men—is most likely due to an increase in male hormones (especially testosterone) relative to estrogen.

These changes can make you feel more negative about your body and your appearance. You might feel that your body, shape, and weight are out of control, which can deflate your self-esteem—providing an ideal setup for Runaway Eating.

So what can you do to ward off or at least minimize these changes in weight and shape? Not surprisingly, our old friends exercising and eating sensibly are the answers.

Join in some aerobic and strength-training exercise. Exercise is an excellent way to stave off weight gain (whether age-related or menopause-related), while improving both your body image and self-esteem. Studies of postmenopausal women with high levels of physical activity show that they have less body fat and less abdominal fat than those who are sedentary, and they are less likely to gain abdominal or body fat in the first place. Exercisers also experience more positive moods than nonexercisers. But this doesn't mean that you have to go into rigorous training; even a little exercise may be of some help. Pre- and postmenopausal women showed significantly better moods immediately after taking a single aerobics class.

Aerobic exercise—activities such as walking, dancing, and cycling that get your heart beating faster and your breath coming harder—helps speed up your metabolism by burning fat, thereby increasing your muscle-to-fat ratio. (Menopause does the opposite.) Because muscle tissue requires more calories than fat tissue to "stay alive," the higher your muscle-to-fat ratio, the more calories you'll burn, even when you're resting. (See chapter 9 for more on aerobic exercise.)

Strength-training exercises—such as swimming, doing push-ups, and weight lifting—pit the strength of your muscles against some kind of resistance, whether it's weight, gravity, water, or even another part of your body. Because it increases your muscle mass, strength training is an excellent way to increase your metabolism.

For best results, your exercise program should include both aerobic and strength-training exercises, done on alternate days. For example, a good plan would be 20 to 30 minutes of aerobics on Monday, Wednesday, and Friday and 10 to 15 (building up to 20 to 30) minutes of strength training on Tuesday, Thursday, and Saturday.

Eat sensibly and often. Eating highly nutritious foods in moderate amounts is always important, but it may be even more crucial during the menopausal years to avoid gaining excess weight. Aim for meals based on vegetables, fruits, whole grains, and small amounts of meat, fish, poultry, and fat-free or low-fat dairy products. Make every bite count! Pay attention to your hunger and satiety signals and try not to eat for other reasons.

A good way to speed up your metabolism is to eat several small meals a day. Your body tends to burn calories more conservatively when you go a long time between meals. But when the food supply is plentiful and your blood glucose levels stay relatively even, just the opposite happens: Your metabolism speeds up. It's as if the body says to itself, "We've got plenty of food now, so there's no need to hold on to every calorie."

Keep the meals small and make sure each includes a high-fiber food (fresh vegetables or fruits, whole grains) and a high-protein food (cottage cheese, nuts, lean meat, legumes, and the like). (The only exception to this rule concerns Runaway Eaters who are experiencing problems with depression and may also be struggling with bingeing or anxiety. If this describes you, turn back to page 194 for a modified plan.) Skipping meals and fasting are the archenemies of a speedy metabolism, so don't engage in these unhealthy practices.

Think it through. Use the techniques outlined in chapter 6 to identify the menopause-related triggers that lead to your Runaway Eating. Then turn to the strategies in chapters 7 and 8 for help in rerouting the negative thoughts and boosting the low moods you may be experiencing.

Estrogen-Related Appetite Changes

Once you reach the postmenopausal phase, you'll have about one-tenth as much estrogen as you did when you were premenopausal—a change that can make a difference in your eating habits. One function of estrogen is to stimulate the production of serotonin, the hormone that signals satisfaction and fullness and tells you it's time to stop eating. So when estrogen levels decline, serotonin can follow suit, confounding your body's ability to recognize when it's full. You can also find your appetite increasing, because a form of estrogen called estradiol appears to help control eating, particularly in regard to meal size. Animal studies have shown that when the ovaries are removed and estradiol levels plunge, food intake increases. But when estradiol is replaced, the normal pattern of food intake reappears. Estradiol increases the action of certain hormones in the gut, especially cholecystokinin, which plays a part in telling the brain that enough food has been eaten. Although more research is needed, the decline in estradiol could be one reason for the weight gain seen in women going through menopause.

Dwindling estrogen may also have less-direct effects on your eating behaviors. As estrogen declines, hot flashes, night sweats, vaginal dryness, difficulty concentrating, sleeplessness, and moodiness can disrupt both your life and your sense of well-being. These additional problems and stressors may be enough to trigger some of those old, unhealthy Runaway Eating behaviors.

It seems obvious that the "solution" for problems caused by low levels of estrogen is estrogen replacement, but recent studies have shown that taking synthetic estrogen may be dangerous, and it's still unclear whether it's safe to take natural estrogen. Luckily, there are ways to increase your estrogen supply naturally.

Exercise regularly to increase estrogen levels. A study of premenopausal and postmenopausal women found that estrogen levels increased in both groups after they took part in an aerobic training program. Plus, more than half of the postmenopausal women had fewer hot flashes, a classic symptom of estrogen deficiency. A different study found that women who didn't exercise had three times the risk of getting hot flashes.

Exercise becomes even more important at menopause, when you lose estrogen's protective effects against bone loss and heart disease. By making exercise a habit, you can do much to decrease your risk of bone fractures, osteoporosis, heart disease, and diabetes. In general, women who exercise regularly tend to have fewer menopausal problems, including obesity.

Stop smoking. Smoking lowers the amount of estrogen in the body, which is believed to be the reason it increases the number and severity of hot flashes and is a major risk factor for osteoporosis. By the age of 80, the bone density in a smoker will be an average of 6 to 10 percent lower than in a nonsmoker, making her twice as likely to have a spinal fracture and 50 percent more likely to have a hip fracture. And if hot flashes and osteoporosis aren't bad enough, smoking also increases your risk of heart disease, lung cancer, breast cancer, and other kinds of cancer. See your health provider to find out how to quit.

Increase your intake of phytoestrogens. A popular way to boost estrogen levels is through the use of phytoestrogens, substances found in certain plants that have an estrogen-like effect on the body. Although phytoestrogens aren't the same thing as estrogen, they can function like this hormone once they're inside your body.

To understand why phytoestrogens can act like real estrogen in your body, you need to understand how the real thing works. Molecules of estrogen are like little keys that float through your bloodstream in search of cells that are estrogen-sensitive, most notably those found in the breast, reproductive organs, brain, and bladder. These cells have little "locks" on their rims called estrogen receptor sites that can be opened only by the estrogen molecule keys. Thus, the cell is able to lock out other nonestrogen molecules until the real McCoy floats by, inserts itself into the "lock," and enters.

Phytoestrogens can fool the estrogen receptor sites because they are shaped enough like the estrogen key to fit into the lock and enter the cell. But your own estrogen is about 400 times more powerful than phytoestrogens, a fact that turns out to be a boon for women who have estrogen levels that are either too high or too low. How does this happen? If you have an excess of estrogen, the phytoestrogen keys and your natural estrogen will become rivals for the receptor site locks. In the struggle, some of your natural estrogen will get locked out and replaced with the phytoestrogens'

BEAT HOT FLASHES WITH SOY

In Japan, hot flashes are so rare that the Japanese don't even have a word to describe them. Many experts believe that this is due to their high intake of soy and soy products, the food that is by far the richest source of phytoestrogens. Studies have shown that eating just 1 cup of soybeans (approximately 300 milligrams of isoflavones) provides about 0.45 milligram of conjugated estrogens, the equivalent of one tablet of Premarin.

Countless studies have shown that soy and soy isoflavones can ease hot flashes and night sweats, two hallmarks of estrogen deficiency, prompting the American College of Obstetricians and Gynecologists to give their official stamp of approval to soy for relief of these symptoms. You might find this particularly interesting if you suffer from depression, irritability, and mood swings, as all of these can stem from a lack of sleep due to temperature fluctuations during the night. And just because you're not waking up wringing wet doesn't mean that temperature changes aren't disturbing your sleep—an increase of just a couple of degrees can do it. If hot flashes or night sweats are affecting your moods, your sleep, or life in general, try eating a couple of servings of soy foods per week in addition to eating a diet rich in fruits, vegetables, and whole grains.

Avoid supplements containing soy isoflavones, however, because an excess of soy chemicals may increase the risk of breast cancer and pancreatic cancer, interfere with the body's ability to absorb minerals, and promote thyroid abnormalities.

much weaker form of the hormone, effectively lowering your estrogen levels. But if you have an estrogen deficiency, the phytoestrogens will add to your estrogen quotient by unlocking cells that would have been ignored. So whether your estrogen levels are high or low, phytoestrogens may be able to help balance them.

There are two kinds of phytoestrogens: lignans and isoflavones. Lignans are found in flaxseed, whole grains, and (in lower amounts) celery, alfalfa, fennel, apples, parsley, and nuts. Iso-flavones are found mostly in soybeans and its derivatives, including soy flour, soy milk, miso, tofu, tempeh, and natto. Herb sources of phytoestrogens include anise, red clover, and licorice root.

Blood Sugar Imbalances

Menopause can also affect your blood sugar, causing it to rise higher or fall lower than usual (or both). This may be at least partly due to fluctuating estrogen levels. Estrogen seems to have a stabilizing effect on fasting blood glucose and insulin levels. And some studies have shown that women tend to eat less during the ovulatory phase, when estrogen levels are high, which may be because blood glucose levels are normalized. But as estrogen levels decline following menopause, some women may find the effect is reversed. One thing is certain: Any tendency toward blood sugar swings will be made worse by eating a diet that is high in refined carbohydrates (simple sugars and starches) and highly processed, low-fiber, nutrient-poor foods.

What's so bad about refined carbs? They're quickly broken down and released into the bloodstream as glucose. And though glucose is a good thing (it's the body's fuel), when large amounts hit the bloodstream all at once, it's stressful for the body. That's because glucose has to be picked up and ferried into the cells, a job for the hormone insulin. Molecules of insulin act like a fleet of little boats that pick up excess glucose and carry it to special "docks" on the cells, where the glucose "cargo" is unloaded. But sometimes too much insulin is produced, and the fleet picks up too much glucose, leaving the blood with abnormally low glucose levels. This can leave you feeling weak, shaky, headachy, and hungry. And because your brain is fueled almost entirely by glucose, too little blood sugar can severely impact your moods, contributing to depression, irritability, and anxiety.

Likewise, high amounts of blood sugar that don't clear as quickly as they should can also wreak havoc on your body. This happens to certain people who develop a condition called insulin resistance. The docks that welcomed deliveries of glucose in the past either take longer to accept it or refuse it altogether. As a result, glucose begins to back up in the bloodstream. The glucose can either rise to diabetic levels (type 2 diabetes), or if the body produces higher and higher amounts of insulin, the "docking" action can finally be completed.

Insulin resistance and high blood glucose levels greatly increase your risk of heart disease by contributing to elevated "bad" LDL cholesterol, lowered "good" HDL cholesterol, high levels of triglycerides (a type of blood fat), and high blood pressure. Insulin resistance shows up more often during the menopausal years, possibly because estrogen increases the effectiveness of insulin, so as this hormone dwindles, insulin becomes less potent. Insulin resistance is also made worse by the increase in abdominal fat seen during menopause and by a diet high in refined carbohydrates.

Ironically, your taste for sweets may actually grow stronger following menopause. Researchers comparing the taste preferences of postmenopausal women with those of men of a similar age found that the women showed a significant reduction in their perception of sweetness. They needed to take in higher amounts of sugar before they could taste sweetness. Unfortunately, this increased taste for sweets comes at a time of life when there is also an increased tendency to store carbohydrates as fat—one reason that many women gain weight during the menopausal years.

TIPS FOR CUTTING BACK ON SUGAR

To keep your blood sugar levels stable and prevent weight gain, try to limit your sugar intake as much as possible. Here are some tips to cut back on the white stuff.

- Put a small spoon in your sugar bowl and limit yourself to one spoonful.
- Be cautious with sugar substitutes. Sugar substitutes are between 100 and 600 times sweeter than sugar. This can make you want more and more sweetness in order to satisfy your sweet cravings. Some preliminary research on animals suggests that using sugar substitutes can actually lead to an increase in caloric intake. Although we don't yet know how this affects humans, it's best not to be led into a false sense of security by relying on sugar substitutes.
- If you really need to have cookies, try gingersnaps, plain graham crackers, or vanilla wafers, which contain less sugar than other cookies.
- Instead of frosted layer cake, try plain angel food cake with fresh fruit.
- Scale back on desserts and prepared baked goods. And be on the lookout for hidden sugar in all its various forms: cane juice, corn syrup, corn sweetener, dextrine, dextrose, fructose, glucose, high-fructose corn syrup, rice syrup, and sucrose, to name a few.
- Substitute fresh fruit for canned.
- Try low-sugar versions of jams and jellies.
- Substitute plain popcorn for candy.
- Experiment with small amounts of cinnamon, cardamom, ginger, nutmeg, and other spices as substitutes for some of the sugar in certain recipes.
- When cooking, reduce the amount of sugar you add by 25 percent and see if the end result still tastes good. If so, try a little less next time until you've lowered the sugar as much as possible without ruining the end product. Lots of recipes contain a great deal of unnecessary sugar.

Eat to keep blood sugar steady. Both the passion for sugar and the difficulty in metabolizing it will be worsened by the ups and downs of blood glucose levels. Your best bet is to keep your blood glucose levels as steady as possible. To do so, try the following:

- Minimize your intake of foods that contain large amounts of sugar. And when you do eat a high-sugar food, eat it with foods containing protein, fat, and/or fiber to slow the absorption of glucose. Also keep in mind that the natural sugars in fruit can elevate blood sugar, so don't eat fruit alone—add some cottage cheese or a spoonful of peanut butter.

- Eat five or six small meals a day, so that you have a steady, gradual release of glucose into your bloodstream throughout the day.

- Eat complex carbohydrates (whole grains, fruits, and vegetables) with every meal and snack.

- Limit your intake of beverages that contain caffeine to one or two per day. Caffeine stimulates the release of insulin, which can gobble up too much blood sugar and leave you hungry, craving sweets, fatigued, and irritable.

- Avoid alcoholic beverages. Alcohol is derived from sugar, and many mixed drinks contain sugary mixers. Together or separately, they can cause blood sugar spikes and falls that increase irritability, anxiety, and poor moods.

Have more fish. Many people who are overweight have poor blood-sugar control, which in many cases progresses to diabetes. But eating fish regularly may help. Studies suggest that overweight people achieve better control over their blood sugar and cholesterol levels when they eat a low-fat diet including fish rich in omega-3 fatty acids (such as salmon, mackerel, and herring). A 1999 study of overweight patients who had high blood pressure found that those who ate one omega-3-rich fish meal a day while on a weight-loss program improved their glucose-insulin metabolism more effectively than those who just followed a weight-loss program.

Some people prefer to skip the fish and just take fish oil supplements. But be aware that taking more than 3 grams a day can cause gastrointestinal upsets and may worsen blood sugar control in people with diabetes.

Water Retention

Water retention (the buildup of fluid in the abdomen, fingers, and ankles), bloating, weight gain, breast swelling, and breast tenderness are common during perimenopause and may be due to too much estrogen relative to progesterone. (As we mentioned earlier, estrogen encourages the body to hold on to water.) But drinking too little water, eating too many salty foods, and getting too little exercise can also be culprits. An obvious solution is to take diuretics, but they can cause a loss of electrolytes, and the bloating returns as soon as you stop taking them. To keep water retention at bay naturally, try the following:

Drink more water. This may sound like adding gasoline to a fire, but if you're not getting the requisite eight glasses (64 ounces) of water a day, your body can become semidehydrated and send a message to the kidneys telling them to hold on to as much water as possible. The result—you get bloated. If you're drinking plenty of water, however, the reverse happens. Your kidneys "relax," and you excrete excess water. It works best if you spread out the intake over the course of a day.

TIPS FOR INCREASING YOUR WATER INTAKE

The following strategies can make getting your 64 ounces of water each day a little easier.

- Always bring a water bottle along, wherever you go, and take regular sips.
- Drink a glass of water as soon as you wake up in the morning.
- Drink at certain set times of the day—for example, first thing in the morning, when you take a break at work, before you go to lunch, and before you leave work at the end of the day.
- If you work at a computer, set reminder messages to pop up every few hours to prompt you to have another glass of water.
- If you can, drink a glass of water with every meal. Otherwise, drink before or after meals.
- When you want to drink a soft drink, have a glass of water instead. For flavor, add a slice of lemon or lime.

There's also another good reason to drink plenty of water: It may help you to lose weight. A study from Germany reported that drinking water can actually speed up the metabolism. The basal metabolic rate of test subjects was measured; then they were given 17 ounces of water (about 2 cups). Within 10 minutes of consuming the water, their metabolic rates had increased by an average of 30 percent. The researchers estimated that a person who drank an additional 51 ounces (about 6½ cups) of water per day would burn an extra 17,400 calories over the course of a year, which translates to a 5-pound weight loss.

Cut back on sodium. For many people, excessive sodium intake is the culprit behind their water-retention problems. That's because water follows salt. The water-to-sodium ratio within your body must always be in balance if your body's systems are to run smoothly. So any extra input of sodium will require an extra input of liquid. (Ask any bartender, and she'll tell you that salty peanuts make people buy more drinks.) It's generally accepted that the more sodium you consume, the more water you will retain.

Believe it or not, you need to take in only about ¼ teaspoon of salt (about 500 milligrams of sodium) per day to stay healthy. Of course, the average person consumes a lot more than that—somewhere between 5 and 10 grams per day. While 6 grams or fewer of sodium is recommended by the U.S. Dietary Guideline Committee, those who have trouble with water retention should probably limit their intake to 4 grams or fewer. Not only will this help ease water retention, it may also help ward off certain sodium-related conditions such as high blood pressure, kidney disease, and liver disease.

Unfortunately, it can be tricky to get your sodium intake down to that level because sodium shows up in just about everything we eat. The best strategy is to check the sodium content listed on the nutrition label on packaged foods. Try to limit foods that contain more than 400 milligrams of sodium per serving, which includes the following:

- Canned meats and fish
- Instant cereal
- American, blue, Roquefort, cottage, and Parmesan cheese
- Salted chips, pretzels, and crackers
- Frozen dinners
- Smoked, cured, or pickled meats
- Commercially prepared noodle or rice dishes
- Pickled vegetables, olives, and sauerkraut
- Salted popcorn
- Salty seasonings, such as bouillon, garlic salt, onion salt, soy sauce, and teriyaki sauce

- Packaged or canned soups and broths
- Salted vegetable juice

Of course, nobody's suggesting that you cut out all the sodium in your diet. (A sodium deficiency is dangerous.) But by carefully choosing foods that are low in sodium and following a few simple rules, you can pare down your sodium intake to much healthier levels.

- Cut the amount of salt you use in cooking and baking by half.
- Don't add salt before tasting the food you're cooking.
- Get rid of your saltshaker, and don't add salt to your food at the table.
- Limit your intake of baking soda and baking powder.
- Stay away from foods that have been preserved with salt, such as ham, bacon, bologna, and sausage.
- Try flavoring your food with the following instead of salt: allspice, basil, bay leaf, chives, cinnamon, dill, garlic powder, lemon juice, mint, nutmeg, onion powder, oregano, rosemary, sage, or thyme.

If you find it too hard to follow these rules, relax them a bit. Your goal should be to decrease your sodium intake, not to take all the flavor and fun out of your food. After trying this lower-sodium plan for about a month, you should have less of a water-retention problem. If not, try to cut back a little more. If you still can't see a difference after another month, excessive sodium intake may not be the cause. But keep your sodium intake down to moderate levels anyway, because high-sodium diets are linked to several serious health problems.

Get regular aerobic exercise. Walking, swimming, cycling, or other aerobic activities can help ease fluid retention by improving blood vessel tone and increasing perspiration, both of which can be effective ways of releasing excess water.

Consider supplements. Although excess sodium is the major culprit behind most cases of water retention, it can also result from too little calcium, magnesium, or vitamin D, so make sure you're getting at least 1,000 milligrams of calcium, 500 milligrams of magnesium, and 400 IU of vitamin D daily. Of particular importance in relieving perimenopausal symptoms is vitamin B_6, which may help ease water retention as well as mood swings and nervous tension. Vitamin B_6 should always be taken as part of a B complex, because all the B vitamins work together. Look for one containing at least 100 percent of the Daily Value for thiamin, niacin, riboflavin, B_6, pantothenic acid, folic acid, B_{12}, and biotin.

Eat more asparagus. This ever-popular vegetable has been used by Chinese herbalists for thousands of years to treat diseases ranging from menstrual cramping to arthritis. It's a natural diuretic; the root and the fresh juice are particularly helpful in stimulating the body to get rid of excess water and sodium, although the young shoots and the seeds have diuretic properties as well. Asparagus is also very nutritious, containing plenty of folate (folic acid), vitamin C, beta-carotene, and potassium. If you have a problem with water retention, try eating a weekly serving of asparagus (about ½ cup cooked).

You can also try adding celery, corn, cucumbers, grapes, parsley, and watermelon to your diet, because all these foods have diuretic properties. Black tea and coffee (used sparingly) may also help ease water retention.

Consider the lowly dandelion. Most of us think of the dandelion as an annoying weed that invades our lawns. But the extract of the dandelion leaf *(Taraxacum officinale)* acts as a powerful

CAN NATURAL PROGESTERONE CREAM EASE MENOPAUSAL SYMPTOMS?

One of the fastest rising stars in the treatment of perimenopausal problems comes from the world of alternative medicine. Natural progesterone cream seems to offer promise, because a deficiency in progesterone and (its flip side) an excess of estrogen appear to be the cause of a host of menopausal symptoms, including anxiety, depression, irritability, mood swings, slow thyroid, water retention, and weight gain. Any of these symptoms can encourage behaviors such as bingeing, purging, restrictive dieting, and excessive exercise. By replacing the missing progesterone and restoring balance to your female hormone levels, you may be able to ward off a tendency to engage in these Runaway Eating behaviors.

However, these effects can be achieved only through the use of *natural* progesterone, not the synthetic kind, such as PremPro or Provera, which can actually increase depression.

If you're interested in trying natural progesterone cream, consult your physician. It's best to get the cream via prescription. Although it is available over the counter, it's impossible to know just how much hormone these versions contain. And avoid creams that contain wild yam extract, diosgenin, or Dioscorea. Though these substances are identical to your natural progesterone *once they have been converted in a lab*, in their unconverted form they are useless to the body as a source of progesterone.

Side effects from using too much natural progesterone cream can include mild depression, sleepiness, lethargy, and breast tenderness.

---

diuretic that can ease the water retention often seen in perimenopause. One study of laboratory animals found that dandelion leaf worked just as well as a standard diuretic, furosemide (Lasix). As a bonus, though many standard diuretic medications deplete the body of potassium, dandelion leaf is rich in this mineral. It's also an excellent source of beta-carotene, vitamin C, flavonoids, and certain minerals. You can make a tea by adding 4 to 10 grams of dried leaves, 5 to 10 milliliters of fresh juice from the leaves, or 2 to 4 milliliters of tincture from the leaves to 1 cup of boiling water. Drink one cup three times a day.

Caution: Dandelion increases production of gastric juices and bile flow, so do not take it if you are suffering from gallstones, bile duct obstructions, stomach ulcers, or gastritis. If dandelion is taken in large quantities (much more than typically recommended), it may cause a skin rash, diarrhea, heartburn, or stomach discomfort. Pregnant women and anyone taking medications should consult a physician before taking dandelion in any form.

THE BEAUTY OF CHANGE

Dealing with changes—whether they're hormonal fluctuations, emotional adjustments, or life passages—is part of what it means to be a woman. The phases we women experience—puberty, childbirth, breastfeeding, and, yes, menopause—can be remarkably rich experiences, ones that should be celebrated and anticipated rather than dreaded or labeled "female problems." Although you may encounter difficulties or stumbling blocks during menopause and other times of change, maintaining a positive attitude toward yourself and your body can do much to keep you happy, healthy, and active. Here's to a brand-new phase of life!

CHAPTER 12

Pare Down
Perfectionism

We live in a world that idolizes perfection. As children, we watched the Cleavers, the Andersons, and the Brady Bunch all loving each other, looking great, and solving their problems neatly by the end of each episode. And now that we're adults, the media's preoccupation with the "perfect mom," the "perfect couple," the "perfect family," and the "perfect lifestyle" has only intensified. Today, there are numerous cable TV channels dedicated just to making our homes look perfect. When faced with all this, it's hard not to feel inferior.

Women are particularly vulnerable to society's pressures to look perfect. Flip on the television, and you'll find endless ads extolling the virtues of the perfect complexion, the perfect head of hair, and the perfect body. The cosmetics industry makes billions of dollars every year selling us on the idea that we can attain these glorified versions of beauty if we just buy the right hair dye, makeup, nail polish, and lipstick. But it doesn't end there. We're also encouraged to try the latest diets, fancy health spas, tanning salons, and cosmetic procedures such as liposuction and face-lifts—all of which are dedicated to the proposition that we can at least approximate physical perfection, if not actually hit the mark. Is it any wonder that we, too, can start expecting perfection from ourselves?

And what's wrong with that? Why shouldn't we try to do the best we can and aim for perfection? Working hard to better ourselves, achieve our goals, and improve our lives are cherished American ideals. Giving attention to detail, going that extra mile, and pushing to "get it right" can be very good qualities. So what's wrong with trying to attain perfection? Plenty—because trying to be perfect is an impossible goal that can be harmful to your mental health and the quality of your life. We're not saying that it's a bad idea to try to do your best. But there is a world of difference between the healthy pursuit of excellence and the quest to be perfect.

WHAT IS PERFECTIONISM?

Lynn, a 45-year-old legal secretary, was known throughout the office as the hardest-working, smartest, most capable person on the staff. She was also the nicest—the one who always brought in bagels, remembered everyone's birthday, and tidied up the kitchen before going home every night. Besides being superefficient and smart, she looked terrific. Her hair and makeup were always immaculate, she had a beautiful wardrobe, and she got her nails done every week, without fail.

Lynn liked to present herself as flawless. Yet there was a huge disconnect between how she viewed herself and how others viewed her. Her coworkers held her in the highest esteem, wished they could be as efficient as she, and continuously wondered what drove her. She, however, questioned her abilities, never quite felt like she measured up, and was terrified of failing. When her coworkers complimented her on a job well done, Lynn had difficulty accepting their praise and tended to focus on one little aspect of the job that wasn't executed perfectly. It was almost as if she were afraid of admitting that she did a good job. Getting upset with herself for her failure to be perfect was somehow familiar. She couldn't even imagine going out to celebrate a job well done.

This same attitude held when it came to her appearance. She was the envy of her coworkers. Despite having had two children, she wore a size 6, was very fit, and could still turn heads. When she looked in the mirror, however, she focused only on what was wrong—her hips were too big, she was starting to get crow's-feet, her hair wasn't doing what it should. She could never allow herself to be satisfied with what she saw. So despite being exhausted, she would go to the gym and punish herself with Spinning class, aerobics, and weight training to get rid of the extra flab that only she could see.

To Dream the Impossible Dream . . .

Perfectionism is not about doing a good job—it's about trying to do an impossible job. Although the healthy achiever sets goals that are within her reach (usually just one step beyond what she's already accomplished), the perfectionist sets her goals so high that she practically ensures she'll fail. Why? Because she believes that conforming to an impossibly high set of standards will prove she is worthwhile. She ties her self-worth to her accomplishments, but she has to succeed completely. To her, anything short of spectacular is the same as failing. Given the impossibility of her goals, it's inevitable that she will fail. And then when she does, she feels utterly worthless and piles on the self-criticism and self-loathing.

Sometimes she'll go right back and attempt to reach the same unattainable goal. Other times she'll set different (although equally unrealistic) goals, and occasionally she may succeed. But success never brings her a feeling of relief or satisfaction—it's more like an avoidance of failure. Instead of being happy with what she's done, she yearns for an even better performance.

Perfectionism is a personality style, not a disorder. It often develops in childhood and is most likely a combination of inborn personality traits; highly competitive activities; pressures from the family, society, and the media; and unrealistic role models. Many perfectionists came from perfectionistic parents and may have felt that their lovability depended on their performance. Perfectionism can also be influenced by one's genes.

Why Perfectionists Tend to Procrastinate

One of the defining characteristics of some perfectionists is procrastination. You'd think it would be just the opposite, that the perfectionist would immediately tackle every project that comes her way, proving how competent and organized she is. But often, she can become paralyzed by her own stiflingly high standards and her extreme fear of failure. Imagine a writer who insists that she turn out a perfect paragraph every time she puts pen to paper, or an artist who must create a masterpiece whenever she takes out her oil paints. The risk of failing is so high that she doesn't even want to begin. If she never puts a pen to paper or opens her paint box, she can't prove her inadequacy to herself or the world. Her motto could be "If I can't do it perfectly, I'm not even going to try."

There are a few other self-protective versions of procrastination. The perfectionist may start a project but never get around to finishing it. Or she may take on so many projects that she can't complete any of them. Either way, she can't be judged if she hasn't finished, and she can simply blame "a lack of time" for her inability to produce perfection. Because of this, perfectionists are often ineffective and unproductive. They may appear to be extremely busy and important, but they actually get very little done.

THE PURSUER OF EXCELLENCE VERSUS THE PERFECTIONIST

Pushing yourself to achieve reasonable goals can be healthy, stimulating, and an excellent way to grow and learn. But pushing yourself to achieve perfection is unhealthy, stultifying, and a sure way to ensure ineffectiveness and failure. Yet how do you know the difference? How does the healthy pursuer of excellence differ from the unhealthy pursuer of perfectionism? The answer has everything to do with how the person in question feels about herself.

At the core of perfectionism is the relentless pursuit of unrealistically high goals coupled with an overwhelming fear of failure. The perfectionist desperately wants and needs the approval of others, and believes that the only way to get it is to conform to an ideal of perfection. She tries hard to be thoroughly competent in everything she does, and she can be very good at focusing her efforts on attaining a goal. But she often doubts herself; even when she's done something very carefully, she wonders if it was done right. This extends to simple, everyday things, as well: Did she say the right things to that client? Does her hair look good enough today? Did she put everything away in the kitchen?

The perfectionist would like to present herself as flawless and hates making a mistake, believing that if she does, others will think less of her. She certainly thinks less of herself when she doesn't do things right. Unfortunately, that happens just about all the time.

HIGH ACHIEVER OR PERFECTIONIST?

How do you know when your efforts to reach a goal have crossed the line into perfectionism? Check out the following chart, which can help you draw the line between being a high achiever who wants to do an excellent job and being a perfectionist who wants to do *an impossible* job.

The Pursuer of Excellence	The Perfectionist
Sets goals that are within her reach (usually just one step beyond what she's already accomplished).	Sets goals that are inappropriately high and impossible or nearly impossible to achieve.
Sets goals based on her own desires.	Sets goals in response to the expectations of others.
Gives herself a range of acceptable goals. (For example, she'll say, "If I do at least 30 situps, I'll be happy. Forty would be better, but 30 is okay.")	Sets absolute goals: Either she accomplishes everything perfectly or she feels like a failure.
Enjoys the process of pursuing the goal.	Focuses only on the result and does not enjoy the process.
Feels happy and satisfied if she succeeds.	Still feels dissatisfied and self-critical even if she succeeds.

KINDS OF PERFECTIONISM

There are several different kinds of perfectionistic behavior, but three are most common. They're not mutually exclusive; you may exhibit elements of any or all of them.

Self-Oriented Perfectionism

The self-oriented perfectionist requires that she herself be perfect. Her own self-image is almost completely dependent on her per-

The Pursuer of Excellence	The Perfectionist
Believes her self-worth is based on many factors, including her accomplishments.	Believes her self-worth is dependent solely upon her accomplishments.
Doesn't allow her failures to affect her view of herself.	Links her failures to her self-worth. (For example, she may say, "I didn't lose 10 pounds in 2 weeks, therefore I'm a lazy, undisciplined slob.")
Enjoys her achievements and experiences a boost in self-confidence.	Tends to minimize her achievements, seeing them as nothing special.
Keeps her failures in perspective and sees them as learning experiences.	Magnifies her failures, viewing them as monumental, no matter how small they are.
Is driven by a desire to achieve.	Is driven by a fear of failure.
Doesn't feel like a failure if she doesn't reach her goal.	Feels like a failure if she doesn't achieve perfection.
Is willing to try new things or take risks, without undue fear of looking silly.	Is afraid to try new things for fear of making mistakes or looking bad.

formance. For example, if she takes a test and doesn't get 100 percent, she feels like a total failure as a person and criticizes herself severely (even if she gets 99 percent). You might think, then, that getting 100 percent would make her feel good about herself, but it doesn't. She tends to ignore her successes and is always on the lookout for her failures. She often dwells on past failures and spends a lot of time thinking about how to prevent future ones.

Self-oriented perfectionism is strongly associated with Runaway Eating. These self-critical traits apply not only to perfor-

DO YOU HAVE PERFECTIONISTIC TENDENCIES?

Few of us are die-hard, bona fide perfectionists, but many of us have perfectionistic tendencies. These tendencies can put us at risk for Runaway Eating behaviors as well as relationship troubles, job dissatisfaction, or low self-esteem. To determine if you lean toward perfectionism, answer "true" or "false" to each of the following statements.

__ 1. I set extremely high goals for myself. (1 point)

__ 2. If I don't do as well as others, I feel I am inferior as a person. (2 points)

__ 3. I try to do things carefully, but I often wonder if I've done them right. (1 point)

__ 4. I always try to be the best, no matter what I'm doing. (2 points)

__ 5. I get really depressed when somebody criticizes me. (3 points)

__ 6. I need to set the highest standards for myself, or else I'll end up being a second-rate person. (3 points)

__ 7. If I can't do it all or do it well, I might as well not do it. (2 points)

__ 8. I strive for perfection in my life. (2 point)

__ 9. If I don't achieve my goals, I criticize myself. (2 points)

__ 10. Being thoroughly competent in everything I do is important to me. (1 point)

__ 11. If I fail in part, it's the same as failing completely. (3 points)

__ 12. I believe that when I improve my performance, I become more valuable as a person. (2 points)

mance but also to body image, weight goals, and exercise goals. Gaining a pound or finding a perceived flaw in the mirror is torture for the self-oriented perfectionist, who will then pour her energies into trying to fix what she sees as wrong. This type of

___ 13. I often put things off because I want to be able to do them perfectly. (3 points)

___ 14. If I make a mistake, others will think less of me. (3 points)

___ 15. If somebody else does better than I do, I feel as if I've failed. (3 points)

___ 16. I'm good at focusing all my efforts toward reaching a goal. (1 point)

___ 17. What's good enough for other people is rarely good enough for me. (2 points)

___ 18. It takes me a long time to complete things because I'm trying to do them right. (1 point)

___ 19. The better I look, the more other people will like me. (2 points)

___ 20. Being less than the best bothers me. (2 points)

For each "true" answer, give yourself the number of points indicated, then add up your score.

Less than 5 points: You're not overly perfectionistic.

5 to 9 points: You definitely show perfectionistic traits; try relaxing your standards a bit.

10 or more points: Your perfectionism is in the unhealthy range. Read this chapter carefully and apply the suggestions. If you don't see positive changes in a few weeks, see a mental health professional for additional help.

perfectionist is at risk for developing anorexia nervosa. She might set a weight goal of, say, 120 pounds, but once she gets there, she isn't satisfied. She resets that goal to 115, then 110, then even lower, never feeling thin enough.

Other-Oriented Perfectionism

The other-oriented perfectionist imposes her own high standards on other people, demanding that they conform to her ideals. She considers herself the measuring stick for the behavior of others, insisting that they do as well as she would do. Naturally, no one ever lives up to her expectations, and nothing is ever good enough for her. She gets angry and contemptuous when those around her don't perform as well as she thinks they should (which is just about always). Her classic line is "If you want something done well, you have to do it yourself."

Not surprisingly, other-oriented perfectionists tend to have difficulty finding partners and have troubled relationships in general. They can be highly irritable and critical and may mask their constant disappointment in others behind a false smile, yet the recipient can tell that they have, once again, failed to live up to the standards of the other-oriented perfectionist. The children of parents who exhibit this kind of perfectionism can feel as if they are never pretty enough or never do well enough to please the parent. These standards tend to be ever escalating, so even when the child thinks that she has achieved something that the parent will be proud of, praise is not forthcoming. Instead, the comments focus on what wasn't accomplished or how much better the child could have done. The classic example is the child who brings home a report card with all A's except for an A-minus in social studies, to be greeted by a parent who wants to know what went wrong in social studies!

Socially Prescribed Perfectionism

The socially prescribed perfectionist believes that others require her to be perfect, and the only way she will be accepted is by reaching someone else's extremely high goals for her (regardless of whether these goals actually exist). She is overly concerned with meeting social expectations, such as looking a certain way and acting according to rigid standards of behavior, although she feels totally unable to cope with such pressures. This kind of perfectionism is also associated with eating disorders and is linked to an all-encompassing underlying fear of failure. Even the slightest perceived criticism from others brings on self-criticism, hopelessness, and depression.

Because of her fear of failure, the socially prescribed perfectionist is also the type most likely to procrastinate and find ways to excuse an unfinished job, rather than risk failure by actually performing a task.

HOW PERFECTIONISM CONTRIBUTES TO RUNAWAY EATING

Perfectionism, a chronic source of stress, can be a major driving force behind Runaway Eating and is consistently seen in those with full-blown anorexia and bulimia nervosa. Someone with perfectionistic tendencies is more likely to respond to society's subtle and not-so-subtle pressures to look and act a certain way. She doesn't want to display imperfections or admit to any problems. Instead, she tries to present herself as the ideal mother, wife, worker, lover, philanthropist, and community activist. This person may believe that part of living up to society's expectations is attaining the "perfect" body—slim, trim, toned, and fit. She may even think that being slim increases her personal value, and being heavy decreases it. She may also believe that losing weight or achieving a certain look is the answer to most (if not all) of her problems.

In an effort to attain bodily perfection, she may diet rigorously, work out for hours every day, purge, fast, or go through countless rounds of plastic surgery. But no matter how much weight she loses or how buffed her muscles get, she never feels satisfied. Physical perfection (and the happiness she assumes it will bring) is always just a little out of her reach.

WHAT YOU CAN DO TO PARE DOWN PERFECTIONISM

To overcome Runaway Eating, you must first control the perfectionism that helps drive the disorder. If you have perfectionistic tendencies, it means that somewhere along the way, you came to believe that your value as a person is equated with your performance, your achievements, or your looks (or all three). The approval or disapproval of others may determine to a large extent how you feel about yourself. This can make you very vulnerable to other people's opinions or criticisms. To avoid criticism, you may have decided to try to be as perfect as possible. But this only increases your chances of failure, interferes with your ability to succeed, and tramples your self-esteem.

Because perfectionism is a personality style, you probably won't be able to erase it from your life completely. But you can begin to think about yourself and your goals in different, more positive ways.

Set goals that are realistic and reachable. Say no to unreasonably high goals that increase the odds that you'll fail and feel self-contempt. What's a reasonable goal? Think about what you've achieved easily in the past, then set your next goal one step beyond this. When you reach this goal, your next goal should be just slightly higher. Trying to shoot for the top when you haven't made the stops along the way is self-defeating. For example, going on a crash diet to lose 40 pounds is an unrealistic goal. A more realistic goal is losing 5 pounds at a time, for a total of 10 pounds, by eating more healthfully and stepping up your exercise and physical activity.

Base your goals on your own wants and needs, instead of the wants and needs of others. Don't let others determine your goals for you or force you to achieve things that aren't on your agenda. If you want to lose 10 pounds because you think it would make you feel better, then let that be your goal. But don't do it because your husband tells you to or because everyone in *Vogue* looks thinner than you do.

Focus on your successes, even partial successes. Perfectionists are great at minimizing their achievements, especially if those achievements are small stepping-stones toward what could become a flashy, obvious success. An important part of scaling back on perfectionism involves feeling good about yourself, who you are, and what you've done. Pat yourself on the back for the little things you do right each day, recognize the small victories, and realize that the kind of big, flashy successes that you may crave are made up of many small triumphs that accrue over time.

Stop focusing on your faults and flaws. You can spend your entire life thinking about what's wrong with you, but that doesn't help you get to where you want to go. Self-criticism is depressing, defeating, and ultimately paralyzing. Realize that everybody has their shortcomings and you're allowed to have them, too. Then focus on what's good about you and how you can build upon it.

Realize that your worth as a person is not determined by your accomplishments alone. Perfectionists tend to base their self-worth on what looks good on paper—grades, credentials, titles, awards, photographs of themselves that show them looking good. But a person's true worth is measured in many ways. Focus on all the things that give your life worth and meaning. How about the quality of your relationships, your hobbies, your creativity, your spirituality? You are not just an achieving machine.

Focus on the process, not just the end result. If you're interested only in outcomes, you're going to miss a lot of the joy, fun, and learning in life. Climbing a mountain is not just about reaching the summit but also about enjoying the fresh air, exercise, wildflowers, animals, sunrises, and sunsets that you experience all along the trail. If you don't stop and smell the roses, your successes will be pretty empty experiences.

Take anxiety or depression as signs of unrealistic goals. When you start grinding your teeth, getting headaches, waking up at 4:00 A.M., biting your nails, or feeling as though you can't drag yourself out of bed, ask yourself if you've set goals that are just too high. Scale back on your expectations. Whatever you're after, it's not worth risking your physical and mental health.

Embrace your mistakes, they're learning experiences. If you spend your life trying to avoid making mistakes, you'll miss a lot of opportunities to grow and learn. Mistakes only become a problem when you don't learn from them.

Figure out what's so scary about not being perfect. Sometimes maintaining an unhealthy behavior pattern (like perfectionism) is less frightening than trying to change. The self-criticism and negative self-appraisal become familiar, predictable, and almost comfortable. But ask yourself what might be so frightening about saying to yourself, "I did a really nice job," "I look pretty fine this morning," or "I'm proud of how I handled that negotiation." Perhaps there was a Thought Myth from way back in your childhood that cautioned against getting a big head or bragging, and you took that Thought Myth to an extreme.

Patting yourself on the back and saying, "Well done," or feeling proud of yourself is a far cry from becoming an arrogant braggart. A large obstacle to success is inaccurate self-appraisal. By learning to appraise your strengths and weaknesses in a more objective way, you can do much to increase your chances of both success and contentment.

DEBUNK PERFECTIONISTIC THOUGHT MYTHS

At the root of most perfectionistic thinking is at least one deeply entrenched Thought Myth. In fact, one of the thought trademarks of perfectionists is all-or-nothing thinking. (See the Thought Myth section in chapter 7 for a review of this type of thinking.) For example, the person who harbors this type of Thought Myth will worry that she's going to lose her job if she doesn't get all fives on her performance evaluation. Yet one mistake doesn't mean total failure. If this way of thinking sounds familiar, realize that setbacks or slipups are an important part of the process of achieving.

When you find yourself falling into an all-or-nothing trap—or into any other type of thinking that involves a Thought Myth—pull out one of your "Challenging Your Thought Myths" worksheets from chapter 7 and work it through. To give you some practice, and because identifying the Thought Myths of others can help you to uncover your own, take a look at the following example. Then use a "Challenging Your Thought Myths" worksheet to find out what's behind it.

Cheryl's Story

Cheryl was divorced last year and felt as if she was ready to start seeing men. But she wondered if anyone would be interested in her now that she was about 15 pounds heavier than when she was single. Old thoughts she hadn't had since she was a teenager came flooding back to her—thoughts like "In order to impress a guy, you have to look perfect, be thin, not eat too much in front of him, give him compliments, and listen to him instead of talking about yourself." Cheryl could dismiss some of these ideas as pure silliness, but the one she continued to cling to was the necessity of being thin. And even though her body had matured after having had two children, Cheryl thought she had to get back the girlish figure she'd had as a teen before she dared to venture out into the dating arena.

Cheryl's thinking is clouded by lots of Thought Myths, but one of the biggest is her belief that she needs to lose 15 pounds before anyone will want to date her. She bases this belief on an old idea from her teenage years that guys always prefer really thin girls. And the magazine articles she's been reading lately seem to confirm this belief. They say that losing weight after a divorce is a great way to boost confidence and get back into the swing of things.

The idea that no one will want her until she loses 15 pounds makes Cheryl feel inadequate and encourages her to focus on her body and her weight instead of other, more important things. It's also a classic example of all-or-nothing thinking: "Unless I lose 15 pounds, there's no dating for me."

After thinking it through, Cheryl realizes that there are also alternative views: She knows that if she goes on a crash diet, she'll probably be miserable and less attractive as a partner. She also knows that she has a great personality and lots to offer besides her looks and that she's not looking for a guy who's just interested in her body.

Cheryl tells herself that dating at 45 is probably going to be difficult and that she shouldn't make it even harder on herself by setting unrealistic goals. Though she knows that getting back into shape is a good goal, she decides that she will do it for herself and not as part of a plan to attract a man. Her goals are separate and distinct: She will take good care of her body to feel good physically and mentally. And she will look for a man who will love her for who she is and what she can bring to the relationship, rather than how large or small her body may be.

PRACTICE BEING LESS THAN PERFECT

Perfectionism is a personality style, one that may have been with you for a very long time. You may never completely rid yourself of the desire to be perfect, but you can reduce the tendency, freeing yourself in the process. To do this, though, you will literally have to practice being less than perfect and be willing to deal with the consequences. For example:

- Instead of setting absolute goals, give yourself a range. For example, instead of trying to accomplish every single thing on your "to do" list, aim for three to five things— then pat yourself on the back for being within range.
- Just for today, go grocery shopping without first doing your hair and makeup. But don't shy away from engaging people. Engage them with your personality, instead of your looks.
- Just for today, try putting forth 90 percent effort at work instead of your usual 110 percent. See if anyone notices (other than you).
- Admit (out loud) that you don't have the energy to do something that is expected of you. Tell your family that

your day was just too hectic to cook, and have someone else go out to pick up subs for dinner.

♦ List five ways that you can say no and feel good about it.

♦ Take a day off from exercise—regularly—and fill the time with something pleasurable like tai chi, stretching, or a massage.

♦ When you find yourself striving for perfection, ask yourself, "What am I afraid of? What's the worst thing that can happen if I'm not perfect?"

The world won't come to an end and people won't think less of you if you're not perfect. Conquering perfectionism means learning how to be satisfied with a job well done, rather than a job perfectly done.

CHAPTER 13

Staying Out of "The Pit"

"The greatest discovery of any generation is that human beings can alter their lives by altering the attitudes of their minds."

—Albert Schweitzer

One thing is certain: All of us slip, trip, and even fall flat on our faces now and then on the road to recovery from Runaway Eating. When life gets stressful and it becomes difficult to manage our emotions, some of us may yearn for the sense of control we felt when following a strict diet or exercising excessively. Others may turn back to bingeing or purging (or both) for stress relief and emotional anesthesia. This is just a fact of life, so expect it.

Sometimes you may be able to resist these urges, but there will be times when you won't. (Nobody's perfect, remember?) When you do experience a slip, the most important thing is to pick yourself up, dust yourself off, and get back on track as fast as possible before the slip becomes a full-fledged relapse. Forget the self-criticism—it just makes everything worse—and don't try to compensate for your behavior (as in "Because I ate two candy bars, I'll skip my snack or eat only vegetables for dinner"). Simply start again. One mistake doesn't make you a failure, unless you decide to apply that label and take it to heart.

WHEN DOES A SLIP BECOME A RELAPSE?

A slip is a temporary backslide into Runaway Eating, after which you regain control over what you're doing. A slip becomes a relapse, though, if your backslide into Runaway Eating remains out of control and triggers even more episodes of unhealthy eating behavior. Below are two examples of the same incident—one is a slip and one is a relapse.

The Slip

When Jana attended a parent conference for the first time with her ex-husband and his new, young wife, she came home utterly depressed and defeated. She headed straight for the refrigerator, ate practically everything in sight, and wound up hanging over the toilet, alternately vomiting and crying. After splashing water on her face, she fell into bed, exhausted. She didn't even want to think about what had just happened.

The next day, she sat down and thought through what went wrong the night before. She refused to get angry at herself or tell herself she was a failure. Instead, she said aloud, "I know this was one of my old ways of handling a stressful situation. Next time I have one of these parent conferences, I'm going to get a babysitter for the evening and schedule a massage at the gym as soon as the conference is over. After that, I'll relax in the hot tub for a while, then meet a friend for dinner at that health food restaurant I like.

That way I'll be able to relax, I'll get some much-needed emotional support, and I won't even have to walk into the kitchen when I get home."

Jana resumed her healthy eating behaviors right away and stayed on track. The slip didn't trigger any other episodes of out-of-control eating behaviors and had actually been a valuable learning experience. Jana now had a plan for handling those stressful parent conferences in a much healthier way.

The Relapse

Jana came home from the parent conference utterly depressed and defeated. She headed for the refrigerator, binged, then wound up hanging over the toilet, alternately vomiting and crying. She thought, "I'm hopeless. I'm fat, old, and ugly and I can't control myself at all. I'll always be a Runaway Eater, so I may as well just give in to it."

The next morning she felt lower than she had in a very long time. She called in sick at work and lay in bed for most of the day. Then she ordered two large pizzas and decided to have a food fest. "It's the only thing that makes me feel better," she told herself. "I'm a foodie—what can I say? Trying to deny it just doesn't work."

For the next week, Jana alternately binged and purged, feeling certain that she just couldn't help herself. It turned out to be one of the worst weeks of her life.

The Warning Signs of a Relapse

As we've seen in the previous scenario, thinking negative thoughts or sending yourself negative, discouraging messages is a surefire way to turn a slip into a relapse. Statements like "I can't do this,"

"What's the use?" "I might as well give up," "I have no control over myself," or "I'm a worthless person" should be taken as warning signs of an impending relapse. They mean that you've lost your motivation, your mood is low, and you're losing control. In the wake of such thoughts, you're at risk for giving in to cravings and unhealthy behaviors, setting off an episode of Runaway Eating. When this happens, it's important to use what you've learned in this book to turn your thoughts around, get back on your regular eating plan, and remind yourself how far you've already come.

RUNAWAY EATING: LINKS IN A CHAIN

To prevent slips from turning into relapses and to keep relapses from taking over your life, it's important to remember that no behavior exists in a vacuum. You don't suddenly binge, purge, or exercise excessively out of the blue. As we discussed in chapters 6 and 7, behaviors are the result of cues, thoughts, feelings, and consequences. These interlink to create what we can think of as a behavior chain. One thing leads to another and eventually results in Runaway Eating behaviors.

Fortunately, there are lots of opportunities and lots of ways to break a behavior chain, many of which we've outlined throughout this book. You now have the tools to control your behaviors! Be aware, however, that it's a lot easier to break a behavior chain in its beginning stages. Unhealthy thoughts and behaviors build on each other and can be hard to defuse. Though it's not impossible to break a chain toward the end, you may find yourself awash in thoughts like "I've already blown it. Why stop now?" or "I'll never change. I might as well just give in." But when you do take back control toward the end of a behavior chain, it's a very empowering experience. It takes a high level of commitment and shows how strong you really are and how serious you are about recovery. Give yourself extra pats on the back for this one.

CREATING BREAKS IN THE CHAIN

Christine started the day on the wrong foot when she hopped onto the scale, weighed herself, and immediately felt lousy because she had gained a pound. It also ended on the wrong foot at 11:00 that night when she binged on a large pizza and a quart of ice cream and then made herself vomit. Are the two incidents related? You bet. But it didn't have to turn out that way. At many different points along the way, Christine had opportunities to use her tools to break the Runaway Eating chain and return to healthier be-haviors. A slip could have stayed a slip rather than turning into a cascade of slips that might trigger a relapse.

Take a look at Christine's Runaway Eating chain on page 254 and see how many ways you can find to break the chain and help Christine avoid backsliding into Runaway Eating.

Once you've brainstormed various ways Christine could break her Runaway Eating chain, turn to page 257. There we share some of our suggestions for breaking the chain, which are detailed in the text below. Take a look and see how this compares with your ideas. There are no right or wrong answers—just different solutions to the same problems.

> ◆ **The link:** Christine's automatic reaction to gaining a pound was to tell herself: "I'm disgusting!"
> **Breaking the chain:** Christine needs to remind herself that her weight is not equated with her worth as a person, and that it's normal for weight to fluctuate on a daily basis by a pound or two.

CHRISTINE'S RUNAWAY EATING CHAIN

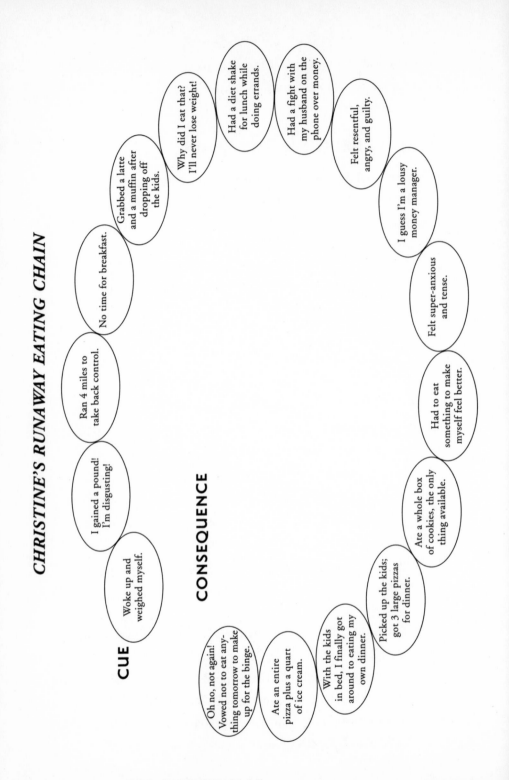

CUE

Woke up and weighed myself.

I gained a pound! I'm disgusting!

Ran 4 miles to take back control.

No time for breakfast.

Grabbed a latte and a muffin after dropping off the kids.

Why did I eat that? I'll never lose weight!

Had a diet shake for lunch while doing errands.

Had a fight with my husband on the phone over money.

Felt resentful, angry, and guilty.

I guess I'm a lousy money manager.

Felt super-anxious and tense.

Had to eat something to make myself feel better.

Ate a whole box of cookies, the only thing available.

Picked up the kids; got 3 large pizzas for dinner.

With the kids in bed, I finally got around to eating my own dinner.

Ate an entire pizza plus a quart of ice cream.

Oh no, not again! Vowed not to eat anything tomorrow to make up for the binge.

CONSEQUENCE

- **The link:** Christine set herself up for a future binge when she ran off without eating breakfast. Because of this, her body had to go without food for about 12 hours, long enough to put it firmly into the binge mode, as she'll find out later on.

  Breaking the chain: It would have been better to make time to eat a healthy breakfast. A less lengthy exercise period might have helped.

- **The link:** When Christine got angry with herself for eating a fatty muffin and drinking a latte, she told herself, "I'll never lose weight!"

  Breaking the chain: She needs to challenge this Thought Myth. Eating one high-calorie snack certainly isn't a disaster or a predictor of her future weight. Christine was overgeneralizing and engaging in all-or-nothing thinking.

- **The link:** Drinking a diet shake for lunch while running errands is double trouble. First, the diet shake is no substitute for a real meal, in quantity, quality, calorie intake, or ability to satisfy. And second, trying to do other things while she's eating doesn't allow her to enjoy her food or recognize her satiety signals.

  Breaking the chain: Christine needs to eat real food in sufficient quantities to feel physically and psychologically satiated. And she needs to sit down and concentrate on her meal when she eats, instead of trying to eat while doing other things like driving or shopping.

- **The link:** When Christine had a fight with her husband later in the day, she took it to heart and made another negative self-statement: "I'm a lousy money manager."

Breaking the chain: Time to challenge another Thought Myth. Christine could tell herself, "Just because my husband thinks I spend too much money doesn't mean that I'm an inferior person. Maybe I need to look over our accounts to see where we, as a family, can cut back on spending."

◆ **The link:** After the fight, Christine felt extremely anxious and tense but just allowed the tension to simmer.
Breaking the chain: Christine needs to do something to relieve her high tension levels. Perhaps she could take a break and go for a short walk or do some gentle stretching exercises at her desk. Or maybe she could make plans to take a beginners' tae kwon do class or get in a rousing match of tennis or squash after work. Simply knowing that she'll get a chance to release some of her anxiety and tension may help her get through the rest of the afternoon.

◆ **The link:** Christine decided to eat something to relieve her tension and improve her mood, so she ended up eating an entire box of cookies.
Breaking the chain: One reason that Christine ate the cookies was that there was nothing else available. By planning ahead and having healthy snacks—things such as cut-up veggies, fruit, whole wheat bagels, and fat-free milk—waiting for her in the refrigerator, she might be less vulnerable to the lure of cookies. And eating regular meals and snacks would substantially lessen her urge to binge in the afternoon.

◆ **The link:** Christine picked up her kids, then grabbed pizza for dinner, an easy food to binge on.

CHRISTINE'S RUNAWAY EATING CHAIN—WITH BREAKS

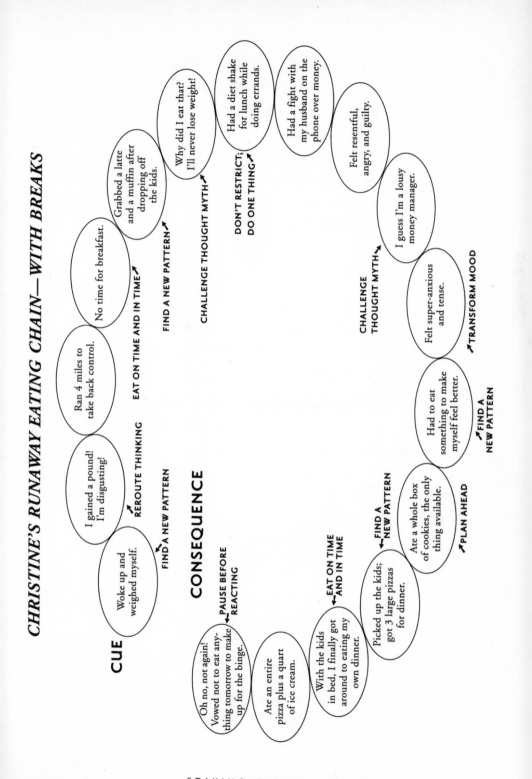

CUE

CONSEQUENCE

Breaking the chain: Getting take-out pizza may have been the simplest way to solve the "I don't have time to cook" problem, but it's not the same thing as a balanced meal. Christine needs to develop a new pattern for the days when she's rushed or stressed. Maybe getting subs would be a better idea—she could get whole grain bread, lean meats, and vegetables. Plus, subs are self-limiting. You eat one and that's it (while you can eat slice after slice of pizza).

♦ **The link:** Christine fed and cared for her kids, waiting to eat her own dinner until after they were in bed.
Breaking the chain: She really needs to eat on time (say by 6:00 or 7:00 P.M.), before she gets so hungry that she's primed to binge.

♦ **The link:** Christine's feelings of horror and self-loathing prompted her to vow not to eat tomorrow as punishment for the calories she just consumed.
Breaking the chain: Even at this point, Christine can break the chain if she stops short and refuses to allow her binge to affect her eating plan tomorrow. By resuming healthy eating with breakfast tomorrow, Christine can keep her slip from becoming a relapse.

Your Runaway Eating Chain

You may want to construct a chain of events that led up to one of your own episodes of Runaway Eating. Working backward from your Runaway Eating behavior, try to determine the thoughts, feelings, and behaviors that led up to it. (Your "Daily Logs for Self-Monitoring" will be very helpful in this process.) Once you've cre-

QUICK TIPS FOR STOPPING RUNAWAY EATING IN PROGRESS

When you're feeling as though you're about to slip into Runaway Eating, try one of the following strategies to get back into control.

- Leave the Runaway Eating environment.
- Use your U-turn cards. (See chapter 8.)
- Practice relaxation techniques such as deep breathing, progressive muscle relaxation, or body scanning.
- Keep your hands busy.
- Spend time with someone whose company you enjoy.
- Repeat your affirmations. (See chapter 8.)
- Repeat your validations. (See chapter 8.)
- Call a friend or your therapist, if you have one.

ated your chain, try to figure out how you could have broken the chain at various links and what tools you could have used to do so. You might also want to make up an "alternative chain" to show yourself what could have happened if the chain had been broken.

LOOKING TO THE FUTURE

Once you understand what's behind your Runaway Eating; once you change the thoughts and manage the moods that drive it; and once you address the issues of anxiety, depression, menopausal symptoms, and perfectionism and you eat regular, nutritious meals, your problematic eating should subside substantially, if not completely vanish. Does this sound like a tall order? You bet it is—but it's also very much within the realm of possibility. We believe that the best way to prevent future bouts of Runaway Eating is to follow the 8-point plan outlined in this book—for life.

IT'S YOUR RIGHT . . .

. . . to be less than perfect.

. . . to live diet-free.

. . . to let go of idealized images of how you should look.

. . . to be loved and respected for who you are instead of how you look.

. . . to base your self-esteem on inner qualities like intelligence, creativity, and generosity, rather than outer qualities like thinness, shape, or weight.

. . . to eat healthful, tasty foods in sufficient quantities to establish and maintain good health.

. . . to stop criticizing yourself.

. . . to love yourself and be loved by others.

. . . to acknowledge your own feelings, no matter what they are.

. . . to make mistakes.

. . . to applaud your own successes, no matter how large or small.

. . . to rest when you feel physically, mentally, or emotionally fatigued.

. . . to take responsibility for your own actions, and let others take responsibility for theirs.

. . . to seek professional help when you need it.

Recovering from Runaway Eating is something like learning to walk. Your family can offer emotional support, your friends can cheer you on, your therapist (if you have one) can give you a rope to hang on to, but you will have to take those wobbly steps yourself. Just like a toddler, you'll fall down a lot. And just as no one can make a baby walk until she's ready, no one can make you give up Runaway Eating until you decide that you really want to become healthy again. But when you do commit yourself completely and feel ready to do the work, you will be able to walk away from Runaway Eating.

We encourage you to pat yourself on the back and reward yourself (in nonfood ways) for every step you make along the road to recovery. Runaway Eaters tend to be generous with self-criticism and stingy with self-praise, so make it a point to give yourself positive feedback, even for the little things. Constantly remind yourself that you are a worthwhile person with many positive traits. Enjoy your accomplishments and savor the praise you receive from others. You deserve it!

Finally, remember that you have rights simply because you're a human being—rights that may have gotten trampled underfoot by Runaway Eating. It pays to review these rights on a regular basis and take them to heart. Make a copy of the list of rights on the opposite page, and put it where you can see it every day.

We wish you the best of luck on your journey toward self-discovery, happiness, and good health!

Notes

INTRODUCTION

p. x   *... up from 42 percent in 1976 ...* Figures based on the National Health and Nutrition Examination Survey 1999–2000.

p. x   *... men aren't doing much better ...* Ibid.

CHAPTER 1

p. 3   *... standards set for the modern middle-class woman ...* J. M. Mannon, *Measuring Up: The Performance Ethic in American Culture* (Boulder, CO: Westview Press, 1997), 88.

p. 5   *... carry their eating problems with them ...* P. Sullivan, "Course and Outcome of Anorexia and Bulimia Nervosa," in C. Fairburn and K. Brownell, *Eating Disorders and Obesity: A Comprehensive Handbook,* 2nd ed. (New York: Guilford, 2002), 226–32.

p. 6   *... more likely than ever to be seeking help for depression ...* R. C. Kessler, P. Berglund, O. Demier, et al. "The Epidemiology of Major Depressive Disorder: Results from the National Comorbidity Survey Replication (NCS-R)," *JAMA* 289, no. 23 (June 18, 2003): 3095–105.

p. 9   *... still lived with at least one parent ...* Jason Fields and Lynne M. Casper, "America's Families and Living Arrangements: March 2000," *Current Population Reports* (Washington, DC: U.S. Census Bureau, 2001), P20–537.

p. 10   *... those in the 55 to 64 age group ...* P. Moen, J. Robison, and V. Fields, "Women's Work and Caregiving Roles: A Life Course Approach," *Journal of Gerontology: Social Sciences* 49, no. 4 (1994): S176–86.

p. 13   *... proportion of divorced to married individuals has almost quadrupled ...* *Vital Statistics of the United States, 2002.* U.S. National Center for Health Statistics (Hyattsville, MD).

CHAPTER 3

p. 65   *... classic study of the effects of semi-starvation ...* A. Keys, J. Brozek, A. Henschel, et al., *The Biology of Human Starvation* (Minneapolis, MN: University of Minnesota Press, 1950).

p. 67   *... nutritional composition of food has an important influence on appetite control ...* C. G. Fairburn, *Overcoming Binge Eating* (New York: Guilford Press, 1995), 74.

p. 67   *... rats given a high-protein, low-carbohydrate diet ...* J. J. Wurtman, P. L. Moses, and R. J. Wurtman, "Prior Carbohydrate Consumption Affects the Amount of Carbohydrate That Rats Choose to Eat," *Journal of Nutrition* 113, no. 1 (1983): 70–78.

p. 67   ... *make you tired, apathetic, and lethargic* ... E. Thomson, "Carbs Are Essential for Effective Dieting and Good Mood, Wurtman Says" (MIT News Office, February 20, 2004), http://web.mit.edu/newsoffice/2004/print/carbs-print.html (accessed July 16, 2004).

CHAPTER 5

p. 97   ... *production of serotonin in healthy women* ... P. J. Cowen and K. A. Smith, "Serotonin, Dieting, and Bulimia Nervosa," *Advances in Experimental Medical Biology* 467 (1999): 101–4.

p. 97   ... *food restriction lowers both levels of serotonin and its rate of production* ... S. Haider and D. J. Haleem, "Decreases of Brain Serotonin Following a Food Restriction Schedule of 4 Weeks in Male and Female Rats," *Medical Science Monitor* 6, no. 6 (2000): 1061–67; D. J. Haleem and S. Haider, "Food Restriction Decreases Serotonin and Its Synthesis Rate in the Hypothalamus," *NeuroReport* 7 (1996): 1153–55.

CHAPTER 8

p. 142   ... *combination of low energy and high tension levels* ... R. E. Thayer, *The Origin of Everyday Moods: Managing Energy, Tension, and Stress* (New York: Oxford U.S., 1997), 107–32.

p. 147   ... *Dr. Robert Thayer* ... *asked 308 people* ... R. E. Thayer, J. R. Newman, and T. M. McClain, "Self-Regulation of Mood: Strategies for Changing a Bad Mood, Raising Energy, and Reducing Tension," *Journal of Personality and Social Psychology* 67: 910–25.

CHAPTER 9

p. 163   ... *half of the women who have true anorexia have suffered* ... D. L. Braun, S. R. Sunday, and K. A. Halmi, "Psychiatric Comorbidity in Patients with Eating Disorders," *Psychiatric Medicine* 24 (1994): 859–67; C. Bulik, P. Sullivan, J. Fear, and P. Joyce, "Eating Disorders and Antecedent Anxiety Disorders: A Controlled Study," *ACTA Psychiatrica Scandinavica* 96 (1997): 101–7.

p. 163   ... *anxiety disorders may be a risk factor* ... C. Bulik, P. Sullivan, F. Carter, et al., "Lifetime Anxiety Disorders in Women with Bulimia Nervosa," *Comprehensive Psychiatry* 37 (1996): 368–74.

p. 172   ... *101 people with anxiety disorders were given either an extract of kava* ... H. P. Volz and M. Kieser, "Kava-Kava Extract WS1490 versus Placebo in Anxiety Disorders—A Randomized Placebo-Controlled 25-Week Outpatient Trial," *Pharmacopsychiatry* 30 (1997): 1–5.

p. 172   ... *Researchers pitted a proprietary brand of kava* ... D. Lindenberg and H. Pitule-Schodel, "D,L-Kava in Comparison with Oxazepam in Anxiety Disorders: A Double-Blind Study of Clinical Effectiveness," *Fortschritte der Medizin* 108 (1990): 49–54.

CHAPTER 10

p. 188   ... *In a study of bulimic patients* ... *depletion of tryptophan* ... T. Weltzin, M. H. Fernstrom, and W. H. Kaye, "Serotonin and Bulimia Nervosa," *Nutrition Reviews* 52 (1994): 399–408.

p. 190   ... *High-protein diets have been shown to depress tryptophan* ... R. J. Wurtman, J. J. Wurtman, M. M. Regan, et al., "Effects of Normal Meals Rich in Carbohydrates or Proteins on Plasma Tryptophan and Tyrosine Ratios," *American Journal of Clinical Nutrition* 77, no. 1 (2003): 128–32.

p. 192   ... *coauthor of the seminal book* Cognitive Therapy of Depression ... A. T. Beck, A. J. Rush, B. F. Shaw, et al., *Cognitive Therapy of Depression* (New York: Guilford Press, 1979).

p. 193   ... *long-term exercisers think more positively* ... J. Dua and L. Hargreaves, "Effect of Aerobic Exercise on Negative Affect, Positive Affect, Stress and Depression," *Perceptual and Motor Skills* 75, no. 2 (1992): 355–61.

p. 194   ... *Studies performed by Barry Jacobs, Ph.D.* ... B. L. Jacobs and E. C. Azmitia, "Structure and Function of the Brain Serotonin System," *Physiological Reviews* 72 (1992): 165–215; B. L. Jacobs, "Serotonin and Behavior: Emphasis on Motor Control," *Journal of Clinical Psychology* 51, suppl. no. 12 (1991): 17–23.

p. 195   ... *a protein-rich breakfast has no such effect* ... Wurtman, et al., "Effects of Normal Meals," 128–32.

p. 198   ... *40 patients with major depression were given DLPA* ... H. C. Sabelli, J. Fawcett, F. Gusovsky, et al., "Clinical Studies on the Phenylethylamine Hypothesis of Affective Disorder: Urine and Blood Phenylacetic Acid and Phenylalanine Dietary Supplements," *Journal of Clinical Psychiatry* 47, no. 2 (1986): 66–70.

p. 198   ... *Twenty-three depressed people, who had not been helped by medications* ... E. Fisher, et al., "Therapy of Depression by Phenylalanine," *Arzneimittelforschung* 251 (1975): 132.

p. 198   ... *73 percent enjoyed a "normal affective state".* ... B. Heller, "Pharmacological and Clinical Effects of DL-phenylalanine in Depression and Parkinson's Disease," *Modern Pharmacology-Toxicology, Noncatecholic Phenylethylamines, Part I.* Eds. A. D. Mosnaim and M. E. Wolfe (New York: Marcel Dekker, 1978), 397–417.

p. 199   ... *effect of omega-3 fatty acids* ... *on patients with bipolar disorder* ... A. L. Stoll, W. E. Severus, M. P. Freeman, et al., "Omega-3 Fatty Acids in Bipolar Disease: A Preliminary Double-Blind, Placebo-Controlled Trial," *Archives of General Psychiatry* 56, no. 5 (1999): 407–12.

p. 199   ... *students taking final examinations who took omega-3 supplements* ... T. Hamazaki, S. Sawazaki, M. Itomura, et al., "The Effect of Docosahexaenoic Acid on Aggression in Young Adults: A Placebo-Controlled Double-Blind Study," *Journal of Clinical Investigation* 97, no. 4 (1996): 1129–33.

p. 199   ... *5-HTP* ... *in a Swiss study of depression treatments* ... K. Zmilacher, R. Battegay, and M. Gastpar, "L-5-hydroxytroptophan Alone and in Combination with a Peripheral Decarboxylase Inhibitor in the Treatment of Depression," *Neuropsychobiology* 20, no. 1 (1988): 28–35.

p. 200   ... *A 2002 review of published studies using 5-HTP* ... K. Shaw, J. Turner, C. Del Mar, "Tryptophan and 5-hydroxytroptophan for Depression," *Cochrane Database System Review* 1 (2002): CD003198.

p. 200   ... *SAMe may help reduce depression* ... G. M. Bressa, "S-Adenosyl-L-methionine (SAMe) as Antidepressant: Meta-analysis of Clinical Studies," *Acta Neurologica Scandinavica* 89 (1994): 7–14.

p. 200   ... *From Italy come two studies* ... R. Delle Chiaie, et al., "Efficacy and Tolerability of Oral and Intramuscular S-adenosyl-L-methionine 1,4-butanedisulfonate (SAMe) in the Treatment of Major Depression: Comparison with Imipramine in Two Multi-center Studies," *American Journal of Clinical Nutrition* 76, no. 5 (2002): 1172S–76S.

p. 200 ... *injections of SAMe were compared with injections of imipramine* ... P. Pancheri, et al., "A Double-Blind, Randomized Parallel-Group, Efficacy and Safety Study of Intra-muscular S-adenosyl-L-methionine 1.4-butanedisulphonate (SAMe) versus Imipramine in Patients with Major Depressive Disorder," *International Journal of Neuropsychopharmacology* 5, no. 4 (2002): 287–94.

p. 201 ... *extract of St. John's wort was just as effective as imipramine* ... H. Woelk, "Com-parison of St. John's Wort and Imipramine for Treating Depression: Randomized Controlled Trial," *British Medical Journal* 321 (2000): 536–39.

p. 201 ... *study with 263 people in which St. John's wort was compared with imipramine* ... M. Philipp, et al., "Hypericum Extract versus Imipramine or Placebo in Patients with Moderate Depression: Randomized Multicentre Study of Treatment for Eight Weeks," *British Medical Journal* 319 (1999): 1534–39.

p. 204 ... *Boosting thiamin levels was found to lift the mood* ... D. Benton and R. T. Donohoe, "The Effects of Nutrients on Mood," *Public Health Nutrition* 2, no. 3A (1999): 403–9.

p. 204 ... *Vitamin B_6 supplementation has been shown to stabilize the mood* ... C. Eastman and T. Guilarte, "Vitamin B_6, Kynurenines, and Central Nervous System Function: Developmental Aspects," *Journal of Nutritional Biochemistry* 3 (1992): 618–29.

p. 204 ... *Folic acid supplements given to patients who were depressed* ... P. S. Godfrey, B. K. Toon, M. W. Carney, et al., "Enhancement of Recovery from Psychiatric Illness by Methylfolate," *Lancet* 336, no. 8712 (1990): 392–95.

p. 204 ... *vitamin B_{12} supplements improved mood and memory* ... I. Bell, "Vitamin B_{12} and Folate in Acute Geropsychiatric Inpatients," *Nutrition Report* 9 (1991): 1, 8.

CHAPTER II

p. 214 ... *less likely to gain abdominal or body fat* ... A. Astrup, "Physical Activity and Weight Gain and Fat Distribution Changes with Menopause: Current Evidence and Research Issues," *Medicine and Science in Sports and Exercise* 31, suppl. no. 11 (1999): S564–67.

p. 214 *Exercisers also experience more positive moods* ... A. Deeks, "Psychological Aspects of Menopause Management," *Best Practice and Research Clinical Endocrinology and Metabolism* 17, no. 1 (2003): 17–31.

p. 214 ... *significantly better moods* ... *after taking a single aerobics class* ... L. Slaven and C. Lee, "Mood and Symptom Reporting among Middle-Aged Women; The Rela-tionship between Menopausal Status, Hormone Replacement Therapy and Exercise Participation," *Health Psychology* 16, no. 3 (1997): 203–8.

p. 216 ... *when ovaries are removed and estradiol levels plunge* ... G. N. Wade and J. E. Schneider, "Metabolic Fuels and Reproduction in Female Mammals," *Neuroscience and Biobehavioral Reviews* 16 (1992): 235–72.

p. 217 ... *estrogen levels increased* ... *after they took part in an aerobic training program* ... J. P. Wallace, S. Lovell, and C. Telano, "Changes in Menstrual Function, Climacteric Syndrome and Serum Concentrations of Sex Hormones in Pre- and Post-Menopausal Women Following a Moderate Intensity Conditioning Program," *Medicine and Science in Sports and Exercise* 14 (1982): 154.

p. 217   . . . *women who didn't exercise had three times the risk of getting hot flashes* . . .
T. Ivarsson, A. C. Spetz, and M. Hammar, "Physical Exercise and Vasomotor Symptoms in Postmenopausal Women," *Maturitas* 29, no. 2 (1998): 139–46.

p. 217   . . . *the bone density in a smoker* . . . M. T. Vogt, "The Effect of Cigarette Smoking on
the Development of Osteoporosis and Related Fractures," *Medscape General Medicine*
1, no. 3 (1999), available at www.medscape.com/viewarticle/408508 (accessed July
26, 2004).

p. 219   . . . *the equivalent of one tablet of Premarin* . . . M. Messina and S. Barnes, "The Roles
of Soy Products in Reducing Risk of Cancer," *Journal of the National Cancer Institute*
83 (1991): 541–46.

p. 219   *Countless studies have shown that soy* . . . A. L. Murkies, et al., "Dietary Flour Supple-
mentation Decreases Post-Menopausal Hot Flashes: Effect of Soy and Wheat,"
Maturitas 21, no. 3 (1995): 189–95; E. D. Faure, et al., "Effects of a Standardized
Soy Extract on Hot Flushes: A Multicenter, Double-Blind, Randomized, Placebo-
Controlled Study," *Menopause* 9 (2002): 329–34; C. Nagata, H. Shimizu, and
R. Takami, "Hot Flushes and Other Menopausal Symptoms in Relation to Soy
Product Intake in Japanese Women," *Climacteric* 2, no. 1 (1999): 6–12.

p. 220   . . . *women tend to eat less during the ovulatory phase* . . . P. M. Lyons, A. S. Truswell,
M. Mira, et al., "Reduction of Food Intake in the Ovulatory Phase of the Menstrual
Cycle," *American Journal of Clinical Nutrition* 49 (1989): 1164–68.

p. 221   . . . *women showed a significant reduction in their perception of sweetness* . . .
C. Delilbasi, T. Cehiz, and U. K. Akal, "Evaluation of Gustatory Function in Postmenopausal Women," *British Dental Journal* 194, no. 8 (2003): 447–49.

p. 224   . . . *a 1999 study of overweight patients who had high blood pressure* . . . T. A. Mori,
D. Q. Bao, V. Burke, et al., "Dietary Fish as a Major Component of a Weight-Loss
Diet: Effect on Serum Lipids, Glucose, and Insulin Metabolism in Overweight Hy-
pertensive Subjects," *American Journal of Clinical Nutrition* 70, no. 5 (1999):
817–25.

p. 225   . . . *a person who drank an additional 51 ounces* . . . *of water per day* . . . M. Bosch-
mann, J. Steinige, U. Hille, et al., "Water-Induced Thermogenesis," *Journal of
Clinical Endocrinology and Metabolism* 88, no. 12 (2003): 6015–19.

p. 229   . . . *dandelion leaf worked just as well as a standard diuretic* . . . E. Racz-Kotilla,
G. Racz, and A. Solomon, "The Action of *Taraxacum officinale* Extracts on the Body
Weight and Diuresis of Laboratory Animals," *Planta Medica* 26 (1974): 212–17.

Where to Find Help

For additional information on disordered eating, or for a referral to a medical professional who can help you with your eating problems, contact the National Eating Disorders Association or one of the other organizations listed below. These groups are dedicated to educating the public about eating disorders and the treatment and prevention of problematic eating.

National Eating Disorders Association (NEDA)
603 Stewart Street, Suite 803
Seattle, WA 98101
Phone: (800) 931-2237 (toll-free eating disorders information
   and referral line)
(206) 382-3587
www.nationaleatingdisorders.org
NEDA provides educational materials to schools, health professionals, community organizations, and individuals.

Academy for Eating Disorders (AED)
60 Revere Drive, Suite 500
Northbrook, IL 60062
Phone: (847) 498-4274
www.aedweb.org
This international organization of eating disorders professionals promotes excellence in the research, treatment, and prevention of eating disorders. The AED provides education, training, and a forum for collaboration and professional dialogue.

Eating Disorders Coalition for Research, Policy, and Action
611 Pennsylvania Avenue SE, #423
Washington, DC 20003-4303
Phone: (202) 543-9570
www.eatingdisorderscoalition.org

This coalition was created to advance the federal recognition of eating disorders as a public health priority, promote federal support for improved access to care, and increase resources for research, education, prevention, and improved training. It provides information on eating disorders via its Web site.

National Eating Disorders Information Centre (NEDIC)
CW 1-211, 200 Elizabeth Street
Toronto, ON, Canada M5G 2C4
www.nedic.ca

This organization provides information and resources on eating disorders and weight preoccupation.

National Institute of Mental Health (NIMH)
Information Resources and Inquiries Branch
900 Rockville Pike
Bethesda, MD 20892
Phone: (301) 443-4513
www.nimh.nih.gov

This institute provides information on eating disorders and funds eating disorders research.

We Insist on Natural Shapes (WINS)
PO Box 19938
Sacramento, CA 95819
Phone: (800) 600-9467
www.winsnews.org

This nonprofit organization is dedicated to educating adults and children about the definition of natural, normal, healthy body shapes and the dangers of excessive dieting and eating disorders.

Recommended Reading
and Resources

CD-ROM

Bulik, Cynthia. *Weight Management with Cognitive Behavioral Therapy.* New Mentor, 2005.

Interactive exercises offer self-paced, private instruction on using cognitive-behavioral therapy to overcome difficulties with weight or unhealthy eating habits. To order, visit www.newmentor.com.

Books

Adderholdt, Miriam, and Jan Goldberg. *Perfectionism: What's Bad About Being Too Good?* Minneapolis, MN: Free Spirit Publishing, 1999.

Albers, Susan. *Eating Mindfully: How to End Mindless Eating and Enjoy a Balanced Relationship with Food.* Oakland, CA: New Harbinger Publications, 2003.

Copeland, Mary Ellen. *The Depression Workbook.* 2nd ed. Oakland, CA: New Harbinger Publications, 2001.

Davis, Martha, Elizabeth Robbins Eshelman, and Matthew McKay. *The Relaxation and Stress Reduction Workbook.* 5th ed. Oakland, CA: New Harbinger Publications, 2000.

Goodman, W. Charisse. *The Invisible Woman: Confronting Weight Prejudice in America.* Carlsbad, CA: Gurze Books, 1997.

Hall, Lindsey. *Full Lives: Women Who Have Freed Themselves from Food and Weight Obsessions.* Carlsbad, CA: Gurze Books, 1993.

Hesse-Biber, Sharlene. *Am I Thin Enough Yet? The Cult of Thinness and the Commercialization of Identity.* New York: Oxford University Press, 1996.

Hirschmann, Jane, and Carol Munter. *When Women Stop Hating Their Bodies*. New York: Fawcett, 1995.

Inkeles, Gordon. *Super Massage: Simple Techniques for Instant Relaxation*. Bayside, CA: Arcata Arts, 2001.

Jakubowski, Patricia, and Arthur J. Lange. *The Assertive Option: Your Rights and Responsibilities*. Champaign, IL: Research Press, 1978.

Kano, Susan. *Making Peace with Food*. New York: Harper and Row, 1989.

Kenyon, Julian. *Acupressure Techniques: A Self-Help Guide*. Rochester, VT: Healing Art Press, 1996.

LeMay, Michelle. *Essential Stretch: Gentle Movements for Stress Relief, Flexibility, and Overall Well-Being*. New York: Perigee Books, 2003.

Lidell, Lucinda. *The Book of Massage: The Complete Step-by-Step Guide to Eastern and Western Techniques*. New York: Fireside Books, 2001.

Mannon, James M. *Measuring Up: The Performance Ethic in American Culture*. Boulder, CO: Westview Press, 1997.

Manton, Catherine. *Fed Up: Women and Food in America*. Westport, CT: Greenwood Publishing Group, 1999.

Normandi, Carol Emery, and Laurelee Roark. *It's Not About Food*. Berkley Publishing Group, 1998.

Pipher, Mary. *Hunger Pains: The Modern Woman's Tragic Quest for Thinness*. New York: Ballantine Books, 1995.

Prochaska, James O., John Norcross, and Carlo DiClemente. *Changing for Good*. New York: HarperCollins, 1995.

Roth, Geneen. *When Food Is Love: Exploring the Relationships Between Intimacy and Eating*. New York: Dutton, 1991.

Tribole, Evelyn, and Elyse Resch. *Intuitive Eating: A Recovery Book for the Chronic Dieter*. New York: St. Martin's, 1995.

Wills, Pauline. *The Reflexology Manual: An Easy-to-Use Illustrated Guide to the Healing Zones of the Hands and Feet*. Rochester, VT: Healing Art Press, 1995.

Wolf, Naomi. *The Beauty Myth*. New York: William Morrow, 1991.

About the Authors

Dr. Cynthia Bulik is the William R. and Jeanne H. Jordan Distinguished Professor of Eating Disorders in the department of psychiatry at the University of North Carolina at Chapel Hill. She is also a professor of nutrition in the School of Public Health and the director of the UNC Eating Disorders Program. A clinical psychologist who has researched and treated eating disorders for more than 20 years, Dr. Bulik received her B.A. from the University of Notre Dame and her M.A. and Ph.D. from the University of California at Berkeley. She completed internships and postdoctoral fellowships at Western Psychiatric Institute and Clinic in Pittsburgh, Pennsylvania. Between 1991 and 1996, Dr. Bulik was lecturer and senior lecturer in psychology at the University of Canterbury in Christchurch, New Zealand. Between 1996 and 2003, she was associate professor and then professor of psychiatry at the Virginia Institute for Psychiatric and Behavioral Genetics at Virginia Commonwealth University. Dr. Bulik's primary research focus has been eating disorders and weight regulation, which she has approached from a variety of perspectives, including laboratory studies, clinical trials, genetic epidemiology, and molecular genetics. Dr. Bulik has published one book and more than 200 papers and chapters on the topic of eating disorders. She is also the creator of *Weight Management with Cognitive Behavioral Therapy*, an interactive CD-ROM. She has served as the president of the Academy for Eating Disorders and associate editor for the *International Journal of Eating Disorders*.

Nadine Taylor, a registered dietitian, is chair of the Women's Health Council of the American Nutraceutical Association. She is also the author of *Natural Menopause Remedies* (Signet, 2004), *25 Natural Ways to Relieve PMS* (Contemporary Books, 2002), and *Green Tea* (Kensington, 1998) and coauthor of *If You Think You Have an Eating Disorder* (Dell, 1998), *What Your Doctor May Not Tell You About Hypertension* (Warner Books, 2003), and *Arthritis for Dummies* (Wiley, 2005).

After a brief stint as head dietitian at the Glendale Adventist Medical Center Eating Disorders Unit, she lectured on women's health issues to groups of health professionals nationwide. She has also penned many articles on health for the popular press.

Index

Boldface page references indicate illustrations.
<u>Underscored</u> references indicate boxed text.

E

Eating habits. *See also* Diet; *specific food*
  breakfast and, 94–95
  do's and don'ts for, 102–3
  eating out and, 100
  healthy, 77, 85–86
  hunger and, 97–99
  meal planning and, 91–92, 95
  mini-meals, 215–16, 223
  regular, 85–86, 93–94
  restrictive, 109
  rules for healthy
    eat according to hunger and
      satiety signals, 97–99
    eat foods you really enjoy, 101–4
    give up dieting, 96–97, 98
    give yourself permission to eat,
      101
  satiety and, 97–99
  serving sizes and, 95–96
  skipping meals and, avoiding, 18,
    94, 216
  sleep and, 177
  snacks and, 95
  times for eating and, 92–96
  unhealthy, 70–71
Eating out, 100
Eating problems. *See also* Runaway
    Eating
  anxiety and, 106
  causes of, 26
  celebrities with, 4, 52
  continuum of, 25–26, 43
  depression and, 82
  emotions and, 47–48
  excessive exercise and, 39–40
  food and
    cultural and societal roles of,
      17–20
    stress and, 18–19
    women's relationship with, 20–21
  incidence of, 5
  medications for, 78–79

midlife women and, 4–6
  personal experience of, 3–4
  serotonin and, 186
  typical age groups affected by, 4
Eating urges, fighting, 154
Eggs, 89
8-Point Plan
  control of life and, 83
  goal of, 76
  managing Runaway Eating and,
    42–43, 75
  physician consultation and, 76–77
  steps in
    alleviating anxiety, 81–82
    defusing depression, 82
    identifying triggers, 80
    implementing regular eating
      habits, 77
    managing menopausal symptoms,
      82–83
    overview, 76–77
    paring down perfectionism, 83
    rerouting thinking, 80
    transforming mood, 81
Eldercare, 10–11
Emotions. *See also* Psychological
    problems
  behavior and, 109–13, 252
  eating problems and, 47–48
  negative, 71
  Runaway Eating and, 27–28
Empty-nest syndrome, 8–9
Endorphins, 193
Energy
  mood and, 81, 142–43
  refocusing, 154–56
  stress and, 16
  sugar and, 145
Enjoyable Eating. *See also* Eating habits
  benefits of, 77
  do's and don'ts, 102–3
Environmental cue triggers, 116
Environmental stressors, 54–55

loss of control over, 28–29
as mood regulator, 144
proportions of, 95–96
regular intake of, 93–94
restaurant, 100
societal roles of, 17–20
stress and, 18–19
sugary, 19
women's relationship with, 20–21
Food and Drug Administration,
78–79, 199
Food cue triggers, 113
Food Guide Pyramid, 86–87, **87**, 91
Fruits in diet, 88–89
FSH, 207–8

G

Gender differences in depression, 182
Genetics, 53–56
Gibson girl, 49–50
Goals
anxiety and unrealistic, 244
of 8-Point Plan, 76
setting realistic, 242–44
Grains, 87–88
Gratification, need for instant, 126
Guilt, purging in relieving, 107

H

HDL cholesterol, 211
Healthy eating concept, 77, 85–86
Heart rate, 16
Herbs for anxiety relief, 171–72
Heredity, 53–56
Hormones
estrogen
appetite and, 216–20
body fat and, 58, 214
decreases in levels of, 211–13,
217
dominance, 210–11
exercise and, 217
menopause and, 207–8

perimenopause and, 82, 210–11,
229
phytoestrogens and, 218–20
progesterone and, 209–13
fluctuations in, 6, 58
follicle-stimulating hormone, 207–8
luteinizing hormone, 207–8
during menopause, 58, 82
progesterone
cream, 229
estrogen and, 209–13
menopause and, 208–9
perimenopause and, 210
stress, 16
testosterone, 58, 214
Hot flashes, 212, 217, 219
Human contact and mood, 150
Hunger
carbohydrates and, 67
dieting and, 65–68
eating habits and, 97–99

I

Imipramine, 201
Ineffectiveness, personal, 127
Insomnia, 19, 177, 193
Insulin, 19, 223
Insulin resistance, 221
Intimacy, fear of, 107
Isoflavones, 219–20

J

Jobs, challenges of, 7–8
Juices, limiting intake of, 88–89

K

Kava (*Piper methysticum*), 172

L

Laxatives, prolonged use of, 40–41
LDL cholesterol, 211
Lentils, 89
LH, 207–8

Substance abuse, 18
Success, focusing on, 243
Sugar
  in alcohol, 223
  blood sugar levels and, 19
  energy and, 145
  food high in, 19
  reducing intake of, 222
Supplements
  for alleviating anxiety, 170–72
  mineral, 170–71
  vitamin, 170
  for water retention, 228
Sweets, 90–91. *See also* Sugar

T

Tai chi, 167
Tension. *See* Stress
Testosterone, 58, 214
Therapists, 138–39, 204
Thiamin, 170, 203–4
Thinking. *See also* Thought Myths
  all-or-nothing, 125
  anxious, 162
  catastrophizing, 127
  destructive, 70
  magical, 126–27
  negative, 158, 191
  overgeneralizing, 127
Thinness
  beauty factor and
    in 1900s, early, 49–50
    in 1940s through 1970s, 51–52
    in 1990s, 52–53
    self-worth, 57–58
    Twiggy, 51–52
  myth, 124
  Restricting Runaway Eater versus, 32
Thought cue triggers, 116
Thought Myths
  anxiety and, 179
  cognitive-behavioral skills and, 123,
    130

examples of, 123
impact of, 80
mental health professional and,
    138–39
overview of, 80
perfectionism, 245–47
personal
  challenging, 128, 129, 130
  identifying, 128
  rerouting, 130–31, 132, 133, 134,
    135, 136
personal experiences of, 135,
    137–40
self-esteem and, 110
triggers of Runaway Eating and, 80
types of
  all-or-nothing thinking, 125
  catastrophizing, 127
  magical thinking, 126–27
  need for distraction or comfort,
    124
  need for instant gratification, 126
  need to be in control, 125
  need to be perfect, 126
  need to be unique, 125
  overgeneralizing, 127
  personal ineffectiveness, 127
  thinness myth, 124
Topamax, 79
Topiramate, 79
Triggers of Runaway Eating
  bingeing and, 106–7
  body cues, 116
  controlling, 114–15
  destructive thinking, 70
  determining personal, 116–17
  emotions, 106–7, 109–13
  environmental cues, 116
  feeling cues, 116
  food cues, 113
  negative emotions, 71
  overview of, 80
  purging and, 107, 109